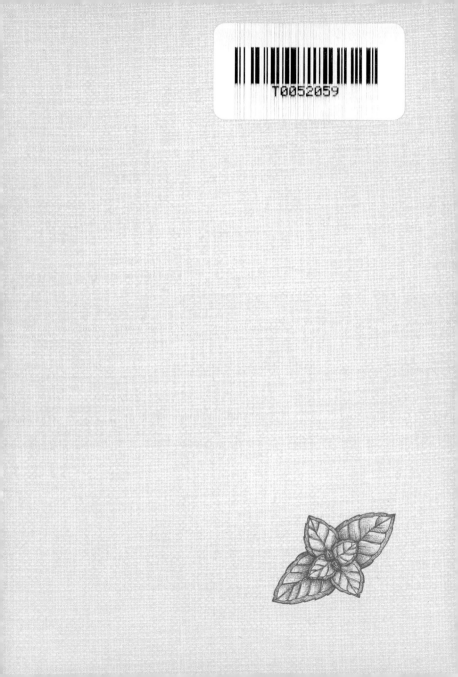

I firmly believe that
by approaching even the
simplest or routine moments
of our lives with focus and
reverence, we create a ripple effect
of beauty and enchantment that
ultimately leads to greater
good in all things.

ENCHANTED
TEATIME

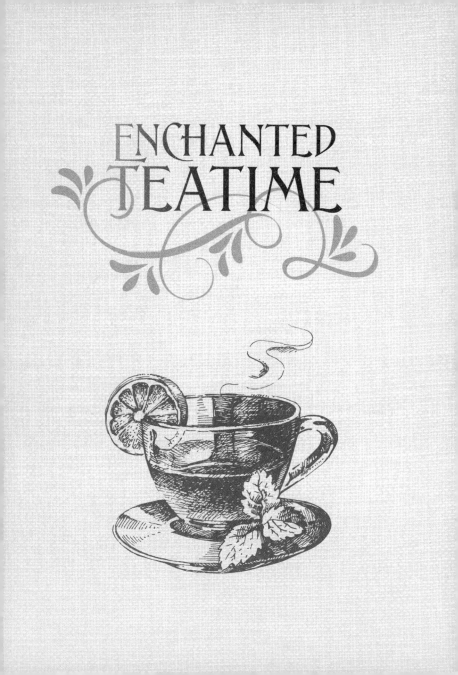

Gail Bussi first discovered green magic as a little girl in her mother's flower garden. After some years spent writing, designing, and working as a professional cook, she decided to return to her first love and obtained qualifications in holistic herbalism, flower therapies, and mindfulness coaching. Today she lives in a small log cabin on the beautiful Eastern Cape coast of South Africa, where she continues to write, teach, and create natural enchantment every day.

Gail Bussi

AUTHOR OF *Enchanted Herbal*

ENCHANTED TEATIME

Connect *to* Spirit *through* Spells, Traditions, Rituals *&* Celebrations

Llewellyn Publications
WOODBURY, MINNESOTA

FIRST EDITION
First Printing, 2023

Book design by Rebecca Zins
Cover design by Cassie Willett

Llewellyn is a registered trademark of Llewellyn Worldwide Ltd.

Library of Congress Cataloging-In-Publication Data
Name: Bussi, Gail, author.
Title: Enchanted teatime : connect to spirit through spells, traditions,
   rituals & celebrations / Gail Bussi.
Description: First edition. | Woodbury, Minnesota: Llewellyn Publications, 2023. |
Includes bibliographical references. | Summary: "Surround every cup of tea with joy,
intention, and enchantment using the inspiring ideas for everyday and seasonal celebrations in this book. Gail Bussi provides ceremonies, rituals, and activities alongside
over 70 recipes for tea blends and treats, as well as insight on nearly a hundred herbs and
spices you can include in your own custom infusions"—Provided by publisher.
Identifiers: LCCN 2023000381 (print) | LCCN 2023000382 (ebook) | ISBN
   9780738772059 (paperback) | ISBN 9780738772196 (ebook)
Subjects: LCSH: Tea. | Herbal teas. | Confectionery. | Baked products. |
   Flavoring essences.
Classification: LCC TX817.T3 B87 2023 (print) | LCC TX817.T3 (ebook) |
   DDC 641.3/372—dc23/eng/20230109
LC record available at https://lccn.loc.gov/2023000381
LC ebook record available at https://lccn.loc.gov/2023000382

Llewellyn Publications
A Division of Llewellyn Worldwide Ltd.
2143 Wooddale Drive
Woodbury, MN 55125-2989
www.llewellyn.com
Printed in the United States of America

This book is dedicated to dear friends who have shared
many enchanted teatimes with me: Lyn and Angela,
now gone into the light, and Caryn, always there
with love. And in memory of my mother, Catherine
Ritchie Bussi. You would have loved this one, Mom!

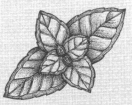

CONTENTS

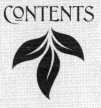

PART 4: TEAS
for Every Day, Season & Celebration

RECIPES

Sweets & Savories

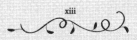

Tea Recipes & Blends

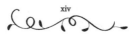

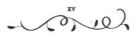

There is something
in the nature of tea that
leads us into a world of quiet
contemplation of life.

Lin Yutang

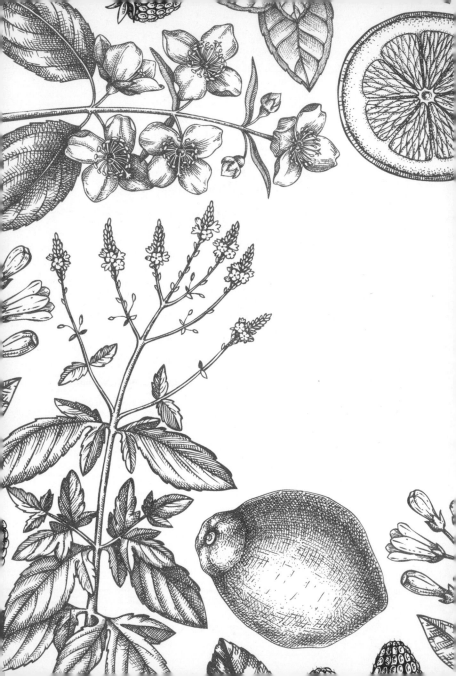

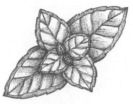

INTRODUCTION

*L*et's have a nice cup of tea." These words were a part of my early life, when tea was not only a daily pleasure but also a panacea for any ills, mental or physical, real or imagined. Taking tea is inextricably linked to my childhood memories of growing up in South Africa, and thus this book really comes from my heart and represents love, memory, and spirit on very personal and magical levels.

My mother's family came from Scotland originally, where teatime, much like in the rest of the United Kingdom, is an important part of daily life—and so it was in our home, where everything stopped for tea at four o'clock and tea parties were a regular part of our routine, either in

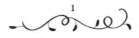

our house or at the homes of friends and family. I particularly remember the Sunday afternoon teas at Aunt Eileen's beautiful Victorian house, sitting around the long wooden table in her dining room. There was a large silver teapot, blue and white teacups, scones, a beautiful bowl of Uncle Bill's old-fashioned roses or hydrangeas, and—always—thick slices of her famous chocolate cake.

In my adult life I have been fortunate enough to travel a fair bit, and I also lived for some time in both England and Scotland: lots of tea shops to visit, some small and cozy ones in little villages, others more elegant in famous hotels in London and Edinburgh. I even worked for a while in a well-known tea shop in London, Teatime near Clapham Common—for me this was like being in seventh heaven, even if there was a lot of washing up involved in my daily work routine.

And always in the back of my mind was the idea of opening my own little tea shop one day or writing a book about tea. But it was only after my studies of green magic and herbalism, and the writing of my two previous books, *Enchanted Herbal* and *Enchanted Kitchen*, that this idea really took shape and form in my mind. Teatime, like so many other simple daily rituals in our lives, can be so much more and open us up to entirely new ways of thinking and being in the world. This is the magic kitchen witches know

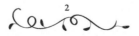

and embrace with joy and reverence: there is nothing mundane or ordinary about our everyday lives and tasks; on the contrary, they can be a portal to new enchantment, hope, and healing if we choose to make it so.

However, the term *kitchen witchery* is not a narrow one or limited to only a few who have chosen a particular path or lifestyle; I believe that it is simply a way of being in the world, whatever our chosen spiritual path or beliefs. We love and honor the natural world and the earth as our mother, teacher, and healer, and the simple everyday rituals and traditions of teatime are a lovely way to access these gifts whoever we are. Tea is for everyone!

Of course, teatime is shared by so many different cultures and traditions in our world—I am thinking particularly of both Japan and China, where their various tea ceremonies are seen as a gateway to greater self-understanding, mindfulness, and peace. This book will share many ideas from these cultures as well as inspiration from folk wisdom to enable us to create our own tea ceremonies and celebrations, either on our own or to share with others.

Perhaps most of all, this book is created with a view to give us all a little sacred space in our lives—time to reflect, to dream, to be. It is in these moments, simple and unremarkable though they might seem, that we can access our true selves and find the magic within. This is the alchemy

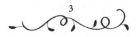

that lies at the heart of our lives—as kitchen witches, we know that our simple kitchen routines of baking, cooking, and the like are a portal to everyday enchantment.

Teatime invites us to step into these moments and find inner nurturing, peace, and joy, which then ripple out into the world and become a powerful force for healing, inspiration, and connection.

This book presents a number of different themes for tea traditions and celebrations, some of which are seasonal in nature while others are suitable for use at any time. There is also comprehensive information about different tea types and their properties and energies, decorating and gift ideas for tea occasions, and, of course, a selection of simple sweet and savory recipes that add to the theme and intention of a particular tea ceremony or celebration.

PART 1

Tea: History,
Tradition & Ritual

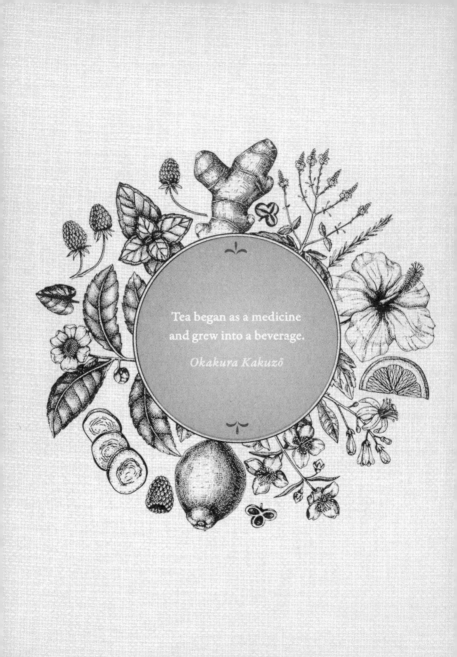

Tea began as a medicine
and grew into a beverage.

Okakura Kakuzō

1

Tea: A Fragrant Ritual & Tradition

*F*rom ancient times, the brew produced by steeping the leaves of *Camellia sinensis* in boiling water was regarded as having many health-giving and life-enhancing properties. Legend has it that the tradition started back in 2750 BCE when the Chinese emperor Shen Nung, who was himself a herbalist, prepared some boiling water for his morning beverage and noticed some leaves had been wafted into the pot by a passing breeze. He was entranced by the fragrance of the hot liquid as well as the sense of well-being and upliftment he felt after drinking this new beverage.

Tea as both beverage and medicine was also revered in Buddhist and Japanese traditions for its ability to

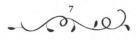

create harmony in both body and mind and allow meditative stillness and peace within the framework of everyday routine. There is a Japanese legend about the origins of tea called "The Eyelids of Bodhidharma." The monk Bodhidharma, also known as Daruma in Japan, came to that country around 520 CE and spent many years meditating in various temples. Finally, after seven years of continuous meditation, he dozed off (not surprisingly)—but when he woke, he was so ashamed of his weakness and lack of concentration that he cut off his eyelids and threw them to the ground. There they took root and sprouted as two beautiful and fragrant shrubs—the first tea plants!

Lu Yu, who wrote *The Classic of Tea* around 750 BCE, said that tea "dispels lassitude and relieves fatigue, awakens through and prevents drowsiness, refreshes the body and cleans the perceptive faculties"—not bad for a simple herbal drink!

Tea took a little longer to reach the West (only after the fifteenth century) with the first advertisement for tea appearing in Great Britain in 1658. It stressed the many medicinal qualities of tea, but for a while drinking tea was considered a somewhat dubious and frivolous occupation! Sadly, tea's growing popularity meant it was heavily taxed, putting it out of the reach of most people and leading to a lucrative trade in the smuggled brew. The tax imposed on tea sold in the American colonies led to the so-called Boston Tea Party in 1773, when men dressed as Native Americans boarded three ships in Boston Harbor and threw all the tea they contained into the sea as a gesture of defiance. This was one of the actions that hardened American opinions against British rule and led to the Declaration of Independence three years later.

Now tea is the favorite hot drink in the world, narrowly beating coffee into that position. I would imagine that if herbal teas were included in these figures, they would be significantly higher, especially in recent years when interest in herbs and natural green medicine has increased so dramatically.

Traditional Teas

It should be remembered that what we think of as being "traditional" teas (for want of a better word) are basically herbal teas too, since all white, green, and black teas start with the leaves of the *Camellia sinensis* or *Camellia assamica* bush, which are themselves classed as fragrant herbs. The different flavor and effects of tea come about as a result of time and place of harvesting, ways of processing, levels of oxidation, and flavor additions (if any).

Tea plants generally are grown in areas of high temperatures and humidity—one of the reasons they do so well in

9

certain parts of China, Kenya, Indonesia, India, and other parts of Asia. Only once the plant is four to five years old will the leaves be plucked, rolled, and treated in heat chambers. Green teas do not undergo the same heating process as black teas; as a result, they are more delicate and fresh in flavor and higher in antioxidants. Black teas are treated in different ways, which results in specific flavors and types of tea.

Traditional Tea Varieties

Tea varieties also vary according to region and ways of cultivation. Some of the most common and popular are:

Green Teas Probably the most widely drunk teas in the world, green teas can have a wide range of flavors and levels of strength. They are very high in antioxidants and are best made with water that is slightly underboiled; if they are brewed at very high temperatures, they can turn bitter and unpalatable.

White Teas While not as common, they are gaining in popularity. They are the mildest and most pure of all traditional teas, with a subtle and refreshing taste. They are credited with many health benefits, including reducing inflammation,

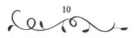

strengthening bones, preventing heart disease, and lowering cholesterol, among others. White teas should preferably be made with water at a temperature of 175–185°F and should also not be allowed to steep for more than three minutes, as they can turn bitter.

Black teas are generally divided into two groups:

Light or Oolong Teas   Earl Grey, Ceylon, Darjeeling, and Caravan are heat processed for a fairly short period of time and therefore lighter in color and flavor than true black teas. Chinese oolong teas are mild and often have a delicate fruit flavor.

Dark or Black Teas   Assam, English breakfast, and Lapsang souchong, which gets its very distinctive flavor from being smoked during the drying process. Chinese black teas range widely in flavor, with one of the best being Keemun, which has a deep, rich taste while still being low in tannins. Both India and Sri Lanka (Ceylon) also produce many types of black tea, with Assam being a classic Indian tea, as is Darjeeling, which has a distinctive and delicate flavor.

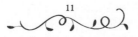

Flavored or Floral Teas   Usually black or green teas combined with other fragrances such as those from flowers, fruits, and spices. This has long been a tradition in China, as can be seen with jasmine tea and Rose Pouchong, which is made by interspersing rose petals with tea leaves during the drying process, resulting in a delicately fragrant cup of tea. Teas are also made with chrysanthemum flowers, orchid blooms, violets, orange blossoms, passion fruit, lychee, and apricot.

The Health Aspects of Tea

Black tea is generally fully oxidised and has a higher caffeine content and greater levels of astringency from the tannins, plant polyphenols that are the oils unique to each plant and carry the taste, fragrance, and health benefits. These tannins contribute to the antioxidant levels, which improve general and heart health and help with digestion. Buddhist monks used black tea to improve their concentration and mindfulness levels, especially when meditating. (Which brings us right back to Bodhidharma and his unfortunate eyelids!)

If you are concerned about the caffeine levels in tea (although it does contain up to 50–75 percent less caffeine than strong coffee), it should be noted that the tannins also found in tea bind to the caffeine and stabilise its effect, releasing it more slowly into the body. Caffeine content in teas isn't governed by the type of leaf or processing method (white, green, or black tea) but by factors like quantity of tea, length of brewing time, and water temperature. Matcha tea is an exception as it has a significantly higher caffeine content, so it probably isn't the best choice for late-night consumption or when you want to relax. Of course, decaffeinated teas are widely available and make a good alternative for those wanting to eliminate caffeine from their diet.

There are other plants that are also used to make teas: in particular, I am thinking of rooibos and honeybush, both of which are native to my home country of South Africa. Rooibos is a bright, strongly flavored tea that is particularly high in antioxidants and offers all sorts of uplifting and healthful properties. It's used to make red cappucino, an alternative to the popular coffee drink; see page 105 for a recipe.

If your compassion does
not extend to yourself,
it is incomplete.

The Buddha

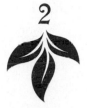

2

More Than Just a Cup

*A*lthough we drink tea as a simple beverage throughout the day, it has also become linked with a particular ritual known as afternoon tea. Some people have asked me where and when this started, and because my family heritage (on my mother's side) comes from the United Kingdom, I know just a little bit about this, quite apart from having spent too much time in tea shops when I lived in London and Scotland!

For the lovely tradition of afternoon tea, we have one woman to thank: Anna, the Seventh Duchess of Bedford, in the year 1840. In those days tea was drunk at breakfast only and then a long day followed with very little sustenance until dinner was served at 7 or 8 pm. Feeling both hungry and fatigued, one day the duchess asked her maid to bring a tray of tea, cake, and simple sandwiches in the

middle of the afternoon so that she and her guests could assuage their hunger and thirst.

This soon became a daily routine, and the custom spread quickly to other upper-class homes in England. But it did not stay there, and within a few short decades "afternoon tea" was a feature of home life everywhere, with guests eating scones, little cakes, cookies, and sandwiches. These simple home teas were rather eclipsed by the very elaborate and elegant teas offered in the hotels of the day, and they are still a major feature of many hotels across the world. At home there was also the tradition of high tea, a much more robust meal that could actually replace dinner and often included eggs, bacon, and pies.

And, inevitably, this was seen as a potential business opportunity, with the very first ABC tea shop opening at London Bridge in 1884. It was an instant success, and tea shops started to spring up everywhere, from the small and simple to the sumptuous teas offered in grand hotels. Tea shops are now a feature of life in most countries, but I believe that it's good old-fashioned homestyle teas that are still the best and most magical of all.

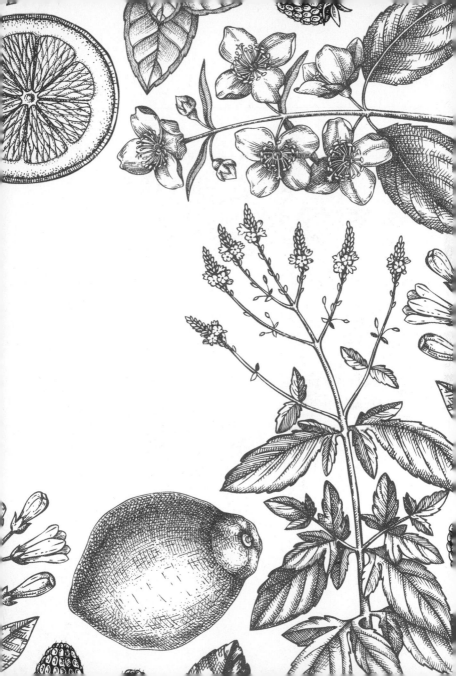

I had always
been here. There was
no need to go anywhere
else. Nothing was forbidden.
Nothing was compelled. Nothing
was lacking. Just being was
satisfaction in itself.

Noriko Morishita

3

The Japanese Art of Tea

have included this because I believe that we can learn much of value from this ancient tradition, one which honors the earth and also encourages us to become truly mindful in the simplest of everyday pursuits, which is ultimately the lesson of tea for us all.

In Japan the tea ceremony, known as *chanoyu*, is almost as old as the use of the beverage itself. It has been seen as an aid to meditation since it first appeared in ancient Zen Buddhist teachings.

It was originally used as a way for the Samurai, the great Japanese warriors, to step away from the heat of battle and conflict and find peace in the moment. The warriors removed their armor and entered the tiny tea houses in a state of retreat and emptiness.

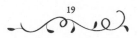

The tea ceremony later became part of mainstream culture and still is today; it continues to embody the Zen ideals of simplicity, tranquillity, and harmony. Visits to the small tea houses are preceded by the removal of shoes and the washing of hands before entering the tea house itself. The first thing seen upon entering is a hanging scroll that usually bears a single line or word of calligraphy from Zen literature. This has been chosen with great care to reflect the mood and intention of a particular ceremony. When the hostess enters, she kneels to prepare the tea, which is done in silence. Either thick or thin green tea is prepared in special tea bowls and beaten to a froth using a tiny whisk of split bamboo before being handed around to the guests.

These tea traditions can be studied in various schools throughout Japan, and many people become lifelong devotees of this art. We can also learn much from this, especially as it relates to finding beauty in the smallest and simplest of moments. Drinking our tea with true care and attention lifts us up to a state of quiet grace and peace.

Lessons from Chanoyu

Obviously the Japanese tea ceremony is something that many people will spend years studying, for the art of tea, as it is called there, is considered a sacred gift, calling, and opportunity. However, I have gathered together a few thoughts about the beliefs and meanings behind chanoyu that hopefully will serve as a guide and inspiration.

- Pay attention to everything.

- Live in this moment, now. There is nothing else.

- If something goes wrong, you don't always have to know the reason. Be willing to allow confusion and upset.

- Simplicity takes both practice and attention.

- Choose what you will focus your energy on today.

- Time and patience are our greatest gifts and teachers.

- To achieve true emptiness and freedom, you must remove worry and doubt.

- Making mistakes is inevitable; they can be the beginning of something new and beautiful.

- Listen to the voice that tells you this is the moment and here is the magic.

- Every day is a gift. (This is a direct quote from Noriko Morishita's beautiful little book *The Wisdom of Tea*.)

PART 2

A Tea Herbal

Making tea is a ritual
that stops the world
from falling in on you.

Jonathan Stroud

4

Making the Perfect Cup of Tea

"*A* spoon for each guest and a spoon for the pot." That was how my mother taught me how to make tea when I was a little girl. She would rinse out the teapot with hot water, add the loose tea (or the equivalent number of tea bags), and then fill the pot with boiling water. This was allowed to stand for at least fifteen minutes before the tea was strained, if necessary, and poured into cups. My mom liked her tea strong—but I have learned over the years that some teas, especially the lighter ones, do taste better given a shorter steeping time, no more than five minutes, and longer steeping can make these teas taste bitter, or stewed.

What about milk, cream, sugar? Traditionally lighter and flower-scented teas do not have milk or cream added,

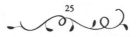

although they may be sweetened with honey, sugar, or stevia. A favorite tea when I was growing up was Russian tea, served in beautiful tall glass mugs set in silver holders, and always with a few thin slices of lemon floating on the top. To this day I just have to smell the aroma of that tea to be transported back to sunny childhood afternoons.

Darker teas are often drunk with milk or light cream, but I must mention that during my time spent in the UK working in a tea shop, any request for hot milk with tea was met with dismay. Hot milk drowns out the flavor of the tea, so preferably the milk used should be cool (not straight out of the refrigerator, though). Some people prefer to avoid dairy, so obviously nut milks, soya milk, and the like can be substituted. In some parts of India and the East, where they like their tea really, really sweet, condensed milk is often added to tea along with various spices. A friend of mine who spent some years living in India told me it was initially something of an acquired taste but ultimately became quite addictive, especially as a wake-up drink in the morning. We won't discuss Tibetan tea traditions, which include adding a few spoons of rancid yak butter to their tea, since it's unlikely many of us have a few yaks in the backyard!

Iced tea has long been a very popular drink in the United States and parts of Europe, although it's starting to catch on in other parts of the world. I love the versatility of iced tea, which makes it a beautiful and festive drink for outdoor parties, barbecues, and picnics. Basically, iced tea is made by doubling the normal quantity of tea used (either green, black, or herbal tea) and then brewing it in the usual way. It is poured into a jug and diluted with water, fruit juice, or other liquid and kept chilled until just before serving, when ice cubes are added and also any fresh garnishes such as flowers, snipped herbs, or slices of lemon and other fruit. Adding some alcohol such as rum or Southern Comfort turns this into an iced tea cocktail, a great drink for special celebrations.

Water for Tea

I am sometimes asked what type of water is best for making tea. Well, the simple answer is water that is as pure and untreated as possible, something that I do know is not always easy to find, depending on where one lives. For example, I live in an area where the water quality is both erratic and often dubious to say the least, and the water is treated with chemicals, giving it an unappealing taste and aroma. I used to make tea using rainwater from a tank, but these days that can also be problematic, given issues of smog, pollution, and so on. Still spring, mineral, or distilled waters are the best and safest alternatives and are

generally easy to obtain. If the only non-bottled water you can use is of dubious or unsafe quality, I would suggest pre-boiling it before heating it for tea.

You can also magically cleanse water by placing a large bowl of clean water in a safe and undisturbed place under the full moon. Leave it there for several hours or overnight for maximum effect. Strain and drink in all the lunar magic! Solar water can be made in the same way, by placing a bowl of water under the sun for several hours at midday. However, it should be noted that this does not render unsafe water suitable for drinking.

Tea Utensils

It's not necessary to have lots of fancy china and other accessories for your tea journey—tea tastes just as good in mugs as in beautiful bone china cups! But there are a few basic precepts that help make your tea experience as good as possible. Firstly, use china, glass, or pottery for your teapot. Cheaper tin or aluminum teapots are not ideal and can leach undesirable chemicals into the tea. The same applies to jugs for milk or cream and also sugar bowls, if you use them.

To my mind, making tea in a teapot—although admittedly sometimes less practical than simply tea bags for each cup—is just magical! There's something about the round

shape that is so appealing and speaks to us kitchen witches of tradition and comfort. Teapots are also practical in that they allow steam to be retained, which in turn results in a stronger and more healing brew, and they make pouring the hot liquid (with care) easier. Tea also retains its heat well in a teapot, especially if you have one of those cute knit or crochet tea cosies—I have several knitted by my great aunt and mother over the years, and although they can seem both retro and a bit over the top, I love them!

The teapot also encourages us to gather round, to create a circle of community and sharing as we wait to sip our tea; this is very much a feature of the Japanese tea ceremony, which was discussed earlier. I love what author Brittany Wood Nickerson says about teapots in her book *Recipes from the Herbalist's Kitchen*: "The teapot teaches us to share…we each may have our own mug, but our tea all comes from the same pot."

Teacups—well, where does one start? I confess to having a great love of pretty floral teacups and have acquired (and broken!) a fair number of them over the years. Somehow I just enjoy the experience of sipping a delicate floral or herbal tea from a delicate and colorful cup, but it's certainly not a prerequisite. Green tea looks and tastes particularly beautiful served in traditional tea bowls made of softly colored glazed pottery without handles or saucers.

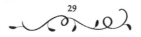

We cup our hands around the warm bowl and allow this warmth to flow through us, body and spirit, just as the tea we drink does.

And then there are mugs—all kinds of mugs: china, pottery, glass...a very practical and viable alternative for everyday tea magic.

But first we need to remember to purify and bless any and all of these kitchen utensils on a regular basis (as indeed we need to do with all our magical kitchen tools). To make a simple cleansing and blessing mixture, combine 1 broken stick of cinnamon, 5 cloves, 1 tablespoon each fresh rosemary and mint leaves (or a teaspoon each of the dried herb), a little finely grated fresh lemon zest, and 1 tablespoon sea salt. Pour a cup of boiling water over the ingredients and stir the liquid slowly and carefully in a counterclockwise direction to help remove any harmful or negative forces or spirits.

Pour a little of the strained, cooled liquid into the cups, teapot, or other utensils you wish to bless, swirl the liquid around with your finger, and say the following:

Cleanse, bless, and protect this teacup
with power and grace. May all who
drink from it always be filled with hope,
beauty, and healing in all things and
in all ways. Blessed be. And so it is!

You can also lightly sprinkle any leftover liquid around the corners and over the working surfaces of your kitchen for additional protection—it smells lovely and fresh, too!

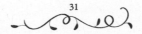

And above all, watch with glittering eyes the whole world around you because the greatest secrets are always hidden in the most unlikely places.

Roald Dahl

5

Keeping a Herbal Tea Journal

am a big advocate of keeping journals. They serve as a meeting place for our thoughts, ideas, and experiences, and can help bring clarity and insight to our days. Perhaps you already keep a herbal or kitchen journal, one that records your experiences with the simple enchantment of your everyday life: in that case, you might choose to simply add any thoughts, discoveries, and experiments made on your herbal tea journey to that existing book.

Alternatively, you may choose, as I do, to keep a small, beautiful journal solely for tea magic. Well, to be honest, it started out beautiful and pristine, but as time has gone on it's become somewhat battered, stained, and worn, but that's also okay. Life is not perfect and never will be—it's about learning and experimenting and growing, and never

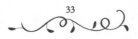

more so than when we are following a green path of herbal and kitchen magic.

In general, I also find it easier to focus on one topic in a journal, and add any material (pictures, clippings, recipes, quotes) specific to that topic. That way our journals can become informative, useful, and also deeply personal, an ongoing source of both joy and inspiration.

There are lots of recipes in this book, for herbal teas of all kinds and delicious goodies to serve with them, but as you go along, you will undoubtedly start creating your own blends based on how you are feeling at that time emotionally, mentally, or physically, or what a particular situation seems to call for. Also, the reality is that often we will discover we don't have the particular herb or plant we need for that recipe or can't find it locally. That doesn't mean we have to pass that recipe by; it just means we have to think a little more creatively. For example, if you don't have any lemon balm immediately available, there are other herbs that offer the same cleansing and refreshing properties, such as mint, lemon thyme, and anise hyssop. Your herbal tea journal is the perfect place to record creative changes and experiments.

Ultimately your herbal tea journey is a very personal one, and your intuition will be your strongest ally in what you choose to use in tea blends, depending on the needs of either yourself personally or those you are preparing the tea for. A recipe is simply a place to start, nothing more. So, as you learn more and go deeper into these green arts, it's very helpful to keep a record of what, when, and how a particular herb or plant was used, either magically or medically. It's obviously also very important to note any problems that may have arisen or contraindications for use. Even if something doesn't seem to apply to you (for example, you are not pregnant), write everything down anyway. Knowledge is wisdom and power.

You will also want to reflect on any tea experiences or ceremonies you may have created or attended. Who was there, how did you feel, and what insights did you gain? This is a meaningful record of magical, spiritual, and practical activity, all at the same time.

When writing and creating your journal, these are some questions to ponder:

- What was I looking for or what did I hope to gain from this tea experience?

- How did I feel during this time? Did I feel more relaxed and able to enjoy the moment?

- What did I learn about myself, about others, or about the green magic path I choose to follow?

- What do I need now? Can I find new joy in this moment and in myself just as I am?

"Just living is not enough,"
said the butterfly. "One
must have sunshine, freedom,
and a little flower."

Hans Christian Andersen

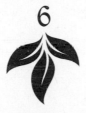

The Green Magic of Herbal & Botanical Teas

*T*echnically an infusion of herbs, flowers, or other edible plant matter is also a tea, but they can also be called *tisanes*, a lovely French word that perfectly captures the delicacy and style of these beautiful drinks. This also distinguishes them from black/green teas made from *Camellia sinensis* leaves. Within each section of this book, you will find specific recipes and ideas for creating your own tea blends or tisanes, but these are just a few basic guidelines to get you started.

Creating Teas, Tisanes, and Blends

Some people have asked me if it's really worth creating our own blends these days, when there are so many commercial tea blends out there—and some of them are truly fabulous,

I must admit. But I still think it's a wonderful idea to mix and match our own fragrant combinations of leaves, herbs, and flowers; in so doing we create something both individual and special. Of course, not all blends work well; I have sometimes mixed up a tea that was truly unpleasant in both aroma and taste, but it also served a purpose in that it was used to water my little herb garden! And if you create a blend that works particularly well, make sure to write down the details in your herb journal or something similar so that you can make it again.

Simple tisanes are made with one kind of herb, leaf, or flower, either fresh or dried. Simply add 2 teaspoons of dried herb (or a small handful of fresh) to a cup of boiling water, steep for at least 10 minutes, then strain and serve. (Depending on the herb, you may choose to use up to 1 tablespoon of the dried plant.) Always make sure the tea is well strained by either using a fine mesh strainer or a teaball infuser. You can also make your own tea bags with commercially available empty tea bags or, as a friend of mine does, create your own using large circles cut out of coffee filters. Simply place a generous tablespoon of the tea blend in the centre of the circle, then gather it together and tie up firmly with a length of cotton string. These tea bags make a lovely gift, placed in a decorative glass jar with a label detailing the contents and the tea's healing properties.

You will quickly come to realize and appreciate the difference between teas made with fresh or dried herbs. Those made with fresh herbs are generally light in color and highly aromatic, with a delicate, subtle flavor. Teas made from dried herbs are usually darker in color and more richly flavored, and they are also often richer in minerals and vitamins than fresh teas—this is a result of the drying process, during which the cell walls of the plant break open, meaning that the water used for tea making can leach more of the goodness out of the herb.

Cold infusions are another alternative when making herbal teas and tisanes, and can be very useful, especially if you are on the road, travelling, or in summer when cooler drinks are more appealing anyway. They are not the same as iced teas. Basically, you make a herbal tea or tisane in the usual way, but you should use a glass jar or small jug with a lid or cover. Place your chosen herbal mixture at the bottom of the jar, then pour over enough hot water to fill the jar. Close the lid tightly and let the mixture infuse in a dark, cool spot overnight or in the refrigerator if the weather is very hot. In the morning, strain the liquid well, then either refrigerate or place in a suitable receptacle to carry along with you.

Drinking these cold infusions is another magical way of tapping into the very lifeblood of our earth and giving us a

whole new sense of nourishment, vitality, and joy. Most of the recipes given in this book also work as cold infusions, but in general I find they often work best when made with fresh or wild-gathered herbs and other plants.

When you make tea blends, you can basically use proportions that work for you, especially if you are adding herbs or flowers to black or green teas. It's best to err on the side of caution initially, though, and not add too much of any one herb since some herbs are very strong in flavor and can be overpowering if not used judiciously, like rosemary and sage. Experiment until you find a blend that is pleasing and enjoyable to both nose and palate. Although many herbal teas currently available often include a large number of different herbs and plants, in general I personally choose to use no more than four or five herbs, flowers, and spices in a particular blend. Otherwise, I feel that the flavor can sometimes become a little muddled and confusing. However, this is entirely a matter of personal choice—do whatever works for you!

All herbal tea blends should be stored in glass, ceramic, or metal jars with airtight lids and kept in a cool, dark place. This applies to both loose-leaf blends and those made up into tea bags. In general, dried herbs have a shelf life of no more than six months to one year; after that time the blend will have lost some of its potency and flavor and should be replaced.

As regards spices, which are also used in many wonderful tea blends, obviously as a rule you will have to purchase these, either whole or in ground form. In general, I prefer using whole spices and grinding them in a mortar and pestle or small spice grinder just before use. That way the flavor is brighter and fresher, as the volatile oils are released. However, it is sometimes more practical to buy ground spices; provided they are stored in tightly sealed containers in a cool, dark space, they can have a very good shelf life, up to two years. Always smell your spices before using them; if they no longer give off a definite aroma, the time has probably come to replace them!

If you are adding ground spices to a tea blend, always ensure the dried spice is very well mixed in, and also that the tea is thoroughly stirred before serving, as sometimes spices can form unpleasant little lumps in the mug.

Please also remember to keep the used herbs, flowers, and other plant material left over from making tea and return them to the earth—scatter them around the base of a tree or over flower beds, for example. However, if the tea blend includes large whole spices, these should be discarded, as they can be potentially dangerous for small birds

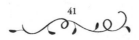

and other little creatures who may try to consume them. I learned this the hard way when I saw a bird almost choke on a star anise pod that I had carelessly discarded in the garden!

A few points about the herbal tea recipes in this book: you will find some specific recipes with each tea ceremony chapter, linked to the theme and intention of that particular tea, and most of these tea blends are made with dried herbs and other additions such as citrus zest, black or green teas, and so on. In some instances the recipe quantities are enough for a single cup of tea, but if you prefer there is nothing stopping you from increasing the quantities proportionally to make a larger quantity of the blend. Similarly, when the recipe is for a larger amount of tea, simply downsize it in proportion to make it more suitable for your needs. Some recipes are given in parts as opposed to specific quantities, as this is also an easy way of adjusting the amount of tea blend you create.

Dosages and Cautions for Herbal Teas

What is regarded as a therapeutic dose of herbal tea? It's another question I am often asked, and my answer is that it's usually a matter of personal trial and error. "Less is more" is always a good rule. Nothing taken in excess is generally helpful, and that includes natural remedies of all

kinds. Just as we wouldn't take twenty aspirin a day, neither would the consumption of ten cups of herbal tea be wise. I always think starting with just one cup, either morning or evening, is a good plan. Notice how you feel. Check in with your body. Do you feel better, more relaxed, more energised, less bloated? Then it's probably safe to say you can continue using that particular herbal tea or blend. Our bodies are always our greatest teachers, and because each of us is such a totally unique being, what works for me might not work for you and vice versa.

Obviously, any immediate unwanted side effects (such as nausea or an upset stomach) are a clear sign to stop using that particular herb or tea blend. It should also be noted that some teas might simply taste horrible to you— it's an unfortunate fact that some herbs and other plants used for therapeutic teas do taste strange, bitter, or like old socks! This can sometimes be overcome by adding honey or another sweetener or incorporating more fragrant herbs such as lavender or lemon balm into the mixture. However, I tend to work on the belief that if you really don't like the taste of something and it makes you feel ill, it's ultimately not going to do you any good!

As previously stated, most herbs and edible flowers are perfectly safe to consume in culinary quantities, which includes taking them as teas; however, if you are pregnant

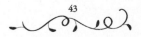

or breastfeeding or have any existing health issues requiring ongoing medication, it's a good idea to check with your medical professionals first. Within chapter 25's listing of each herb and plant used for tea, you will find information about any contraindications for using that particular plant.

You may have to purchase some of the flowers and herbs since obviously we are unlikely to be able to grow everything we need. If you are lucky enough to have some wonderful farmers markets in your area, as I am, then this should be easy and is also a good way of learning and sharing a little more green magic. As far as flowers go, please do not use flowers that have been grown for commercial purposes, unless you are sure of how they were cultivated and what, if any, sprays or insecticides were used on them.

Foraging for Tea Plants

Perhaps you would like to forage for some suitable tea herbs and plants, and that is truly a magical way to find and connect with your own personal favorites. However, there are a few commonsense rules to follow when doing this!

- Firstly, make sure you know what plant you are actually harvesting—many plants look remarkably similar, and one may be healing while the other may be horribly poisonous! Invest in a good guide to the wild plants of a particular area.

- Make sure you are allowed to forage/collect plants in a particular place—there are often rules about what you can gather in the wild and where, and obviously you don't want to be caught trespassing on private land.

- Don't gather plants from obviously polluted areas near busy roads and highways, beside stagnant or contaminated bodies of water, or within areas of heavy industry.

- Never take too much of any one plant—at most no more than one-third. Never pull up a plant by its roots unless you are planning to use the root.

- If you are foraging in the wild, practice normal safety precautions as regards weather and other potential problems that may arise. If you are on your own, make sure someone knows where you are and that you can reach help on your phone if need be.

Some Simple Herbal Tea Remedies for Common Ailments

Please note this list is just a very basic outline; it does not replace proper medical advice on any level, particularly if you suffer from any chronic conditions, are taking

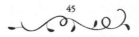

prescription medication, or are pregnant or breastfeeding. Also, please get medical advice before giving herbal remedies, including teas, to children under the age of five.

Colds and Fevers elderflower, mint, yarrow, chamomile, eucalyptus, ginger, rooibos, echinacea, bergamot, green tea

Depression, Anxiety, and Stress lavender, rosemary, skullcap, vervain, geranium, lemon balm, jasmine, St. John's wort, chamomile, basil

Digestive Issues peppermint, fennel seed, caraway, dill, lemon verbena, lemon balm, bergamot, cinnamon

Eczema Caused by Stress and Nervous Tension nettle, geranium, dandelion, borage, chamomile

Hay Fever hyssop, lavender, thyme, bergamot, chamomile, elderflower

Headaches feverfew, lavender, valerian, skullcap, catnip, ginger

Heart and Circulatory Issues (these must always be diagnosed and treated by health professionals!) dandelion, motherwort, evening primrose, lemon balm, flax seeds

Insomnia   hops, chamomile, linden, catnip, mugwort, California poppy, passionflower, thyme

Kidney and Urinary Problems   fennel, yarrow, dandelion, blackberry leaves, cardamom, nettle

Menstrual Issues   calendula, sage, yarrow, chamomile, mugwort, geranium, oregano, clover, parsley, borage

Muscles and Joints   burdock, ginger, nettle, oregano, yarrow

Nausea and Vomiting   basil, ginger, peppermint, bergamot, lemon balm, rooibos, turmeric

Rheumatism/Arthritis   ginger, nettle, thyme, gotu kola, catnip, comfrey, rosemary

Sinusitis   basil, elderflower, majoram, peppermint

Tonics for General Health and Well-Being   borage, cornflower, parsley, nettle, thyme, echinacea, basil, green tea, rooibos

One should lie empty, open, choiceless as a beach——waiting for a gift from the sea...

Anne Morrow Lindbergh

Creating Personal Tea Rituals & Ceremonies

We usually plan and create ceremonies around the special events and seasons of our lives, but each and every teatime, no matter how simple, can be a celebration of peace and joy. It serves as a portal leading us to a quieter and more reflective way of being; this is particularly important in times of change or difficulty so that we are reminded of our own innate magic and strength and in doing so are able to see a clearer path forward. Plus, it's just plain fun to share and enjoy the moment as it is, as we are! I firmly believe that by approaching even the simplest or routine moments of our lives with focus and reverence, we create a ripple effect of beauty and enchantment that ultimately leads to greater good in all things.

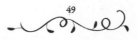

In these times, which can be fragmented, stressful, and confusing, we need everyday rituals more than ever, for they have the universal ability to ground and calm us, whoever we are and wherever we may live.

Every time we make and drink a cup of tea, we are engaging in a simple ritual and opening up to all of our senses as we do so. No matter where we are, what our situation, or how we are feeling, we can use this time to soften and still our bodies and minds, and become aware of the infinite magic that exists in the simplest of moments. As we raise the cup to our lips for the first sip, we step through the doorway into a new realm of quiet consciousness. We can pause and consider what it is we want to take away from these peaceful moments and reflect on what different choices we might need to make in our life. If we are using a tea blend that is linked to some particular emotion or other issue, this is the time to quietly reflect on that too and allow our emotions to be as they are.

However, whatever your intention with a particular teatime may be and whether you are alone or sharing it with others, here are a few additional ideas for creating memorable and magical ceremonies. The initial step is to focus on what it is we need to create, honor, or take away from this ceremony, either individually or as a group. Intention is an important part of any ritual and gives it both meaning and substance. Perhaps the intention is just to chill out and enjoy being in each other's company, which is fine too!

Then comes the ceremony or ritual itself; you will find some more ideas for specific tea rituals later in the book. The main thing is that we remain present, open, and relaxed as we sip our tea and enjoy being in the moment.

First, gather your tea items together (cups, teapot, tea bags, foods you will be serving, and so on). Arrange them on a suitable table or other surface. Light an incense stick or scented candle—I suggest lavender (for peaceful and loving energies), sage (for cleansing and protecting the space), or rosemary (for healing, clarity of thought, and healthy communication).

In addition, I often add crystals to the tea table that are appropriate for the ceremony's theme and intention. Please note that crystals should not be added to teas or other liquids since some may dissolve in liquid or leach harmful chemicals into water. They should be placed around your teacups or on any suitable surface.

Rose Quartz love, peace, and remembering those who have passed on

Turquoise healing and courage

Citrine setting intentions, confidence, and friendship

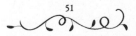

Amethyst creating a calm and soothing
atmosphere, self-knowledge, and wisdom

Clear Quartz suitable for all ceremonies and
occasions and is particularly useful for energy
work and clarity of purpose

Moonstone this beautiful stone is aptly named,
for it is linked to moon energies of healing,
intuition, and magic

Apart from the incense ideas given above, essential oils also add to the spirit and enchantment of the occasion and can be added to oil burners or diffusers. Citrus oils such as lemon or bergamot create a happy and bright vibe, while rose geranium is both relaxing and uplifting for joyful gatherings. Again, please note that essential oils should not be ingested and should not be added to any beverages.

For a simple tea ritual, either alone or as a group, ground yourself by placing your feet squarely on the ground (or earth if you are outside) and hold your arms above your head. Gradually feel a ray of bright light moving from the top of your head down through your body and into the earth below. Say the following words:

This time is sacred—a time apart, a time of
healing and harmony. May I experience its joy
and peace and carry that forward today and in
all days to come. Blessings be to all, and so it is!

If you or others have particular intentions for this time
or people you wish to remember and honor, this is an
opportunity to speak and share these feelings.

For a more in-depth ritual, you might choose to create
a circle of safety and connection. Start this by grounding
and centering your energies, either on your own or as part
of the group.

Standing with arms extended, palms open and down,
turn first to the east and say:

Air, we honor you. Guard and guide
our breath and being. Allow us to fly
high and find our true wings.

Then turn to the south and say:

Fire, you bring light and transformation to
us and our world. Help us burn away what
is past, what no longer serves us, and give us
courage to rise to a new and bright dawn.

Then turn to the west and say:

Water, allow your wisdom to flow through us,
filling us with your sacred and healing energy.
We need your mystery, your depth, and your
compassion to heal our world and ourselves.

Then turn to the north and say:

Earth, you are our home, our mother,
our greatest teacher. Without you we
are nothing. May we truly grow and
flourish as part of your green web of life,
healing, and protection for all beings.

End this opening circle with the following words:

May this ritual and this circle draw all
in to that which is holy, that which is
blessed. May our hearts be open to love,
magic, and the gifts we share in these
moments. Blessed be. And so it is!

When you make and serve the tea, stir it gently three times (the magical number!) in a clockwise direction: this will infuse the brew with positive energies such as health, joy, and prosperity. If you need protection against negative forces or energies that seem to be having an unhealthy impact on your life, you can follow this by stirring your tea slowly in a counterclockwise direction three times. All who are present for the tea ritual should slowly breathe and count to ten before starting to drink their tea.

After the tea ceremony, close the circle by turning in the opposite direction and thanking each of the spirits in turn for being present. Then lower the arms and turn the palms down as a sign that the ceremony is concluded.

And, finally, it's always good to acknowledge what we have just enjoyed and shared, either singly or together— what have we learned in these moments, what emotions came up for us, what have we shared? If candles or incense have been lit, we can blow them out, thoughtfully and carefully, while saying a simple grace or offering some specific intentions.

Some Other Simple Ritual Ideas and Invocations

Every day brings us something to celebrate, something to remember, and possibly something we need to work through on an emotional or physical level. We can use the simplest tea ceremony as a portal to finding greater balance and joy—that is the magic of tea, which is contained not only in its healthful properties, but in the fact that stopping to drink our tea in a mindful way shifts our focus magically and profoundly. As we drink the liquid, we are being filled with its magic, inside and out.

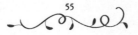

For a simple tea ritual, brew your chosen cup of tea and stand or sit quietly for a few moments. Stir the tea three times in a counterclockwise direction to remove any negativity that may be lurking, and then three times in a clockwise direction to invite positive and magical energies into your life.

- *When you are facing a big decision and need clarity and direction*: Close your eyes and say: "My heart and mind are open as I find the wisdom I need to make strong and healthy decisions."
  TEAS: sage, cornflower, peppermint, rooibos, lemon

- *When you have financial problems and lack in your life*: "I know I am abundant in all aspects of my life, even if I am fearful right now; what I need will always come to me in the right time, and I now choose hope and joy over fear."
  TEAS: thyme, cinnamon, green

- *Anxiety and stressful situations of any kind*: "All will be well—this I trust, as I invite the spirits of hope and confidence; I am peaceful, calm, and clear, and will remain so."
  TEAS: rose, lavender, chamomile, rosemary

- *When we are anxious about love or feeling its lack in our lives*: "Love is at the heart of my being, and so I am never without it, even when I feel alone; it is there and will be made manifest in the right time and season."
  TEAS: lemon balm, rose, geranium, jasmine, vanilla, raspberry leaf, white

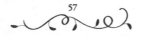

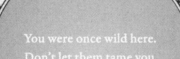

You were once wild here.
Don't let them tame you.

Isadora Duncan

8

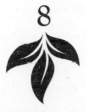

Creating Your Herbal Tea Garden

This is not intended to be an in-depth guide to herb gardening—space does not permit! If you are starting a herb garden from scratch, I suggest you buy a good basic herb gardening book, preferably one that is applicable to your geographic region. However, if you are starting a herb garden, here are a few ideas.

Starting Small

For a first herb garden, start small and keep it simple. Herbs are infinitely interesting and varied, and it's possible to get carried away and plant too many at any one time! I would suggest no more than 10–12 herbs in the beginning, and by happy chance most of these are also part of the herbal tea apothecary, too!

The plants I suggest are parsley, mint (in its own pot, of course), rosemary, thyme, lavender (always, no herb garden is complete without it), chives, holy basil, lemon balm, chamomile, dill, borage, and scented geranium. With these you can do all sort of wonderful things in the kitchen and beyond. Of course, there are many different varieties of each of these herbs, too, so you will probably quickly find your own personal favorites. I, for example, would not want to be without lemon thyme or French lavender (as opposed to the more commonly available English variety).

Gardening is really a matter of trial and error—some plants grow and flourish with a will, while others are more temperamental. (I can say this as one who has experienced some major garden catastrophes over the years!) If the majority of the herbs you are growing are going to be used for tea or culinary purposes, please remember that a sunny area is always the best; herbs generally thrive in sun, and the warmth brings out the full flavor of the volatile oils in plants such as cilantro, rosemary, basil, and thyme.

In France (and likely other parts of medieval Europe) monasteries always had what was called a monk's garden, situated in a bright and sunny spot close to the kitchen door so that the monk in charge of the kitchens just had to step outside to pluck a few fresh herbs to add to the evening meal or whatever else he was making. It's a lovely idea and a good one to emulate if you have limited space since such a garden need only be a few feet square or round in size.

Additional Ideas for Your Tea Garden

If you already have a herb garden, you probably have most of what you need for a good herbal tea repertoire because herbs are such infinitely versatile plants and have such a wide range of uses. The traditional herbs we generally choose to grow are also the most useful ones when it comes to tea; I am thinking of lavender, mint, thyme, and so on. If you don't already have them in your garden, may I suggest growing some scented geranium, both the rose and lemon-scented varieties? Also, a small bay tree, which grows well in large pots, too, as do the smaller varieties of lemon trees.

However, you also need to consider growing nasturtiums, marigolds, chamomile, dandelions (if they are not already part of your garden), borage, fennel, valerian, and some of the less common herb varieties, which can be enormously useful in creating teas and other herbal mixtures.

Larger plants to consider for your garden are jasmine, hibiscus, lemon verbena, and raspberry (which doesn't like being confined to a container or pot). Roses are an essential for any garden, and the variety available these days is

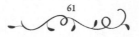

truly amazing; in terms of herbal teas, though, you obviously need to choose highly fragrant varieties that will taste wonderful fresh and also hold up to being dried. I have sometimes tasted dried rose petals that no longer had any flavor or fragrance at all, possibly as a result of being dried incorrectly or kept too long.

Herb Gardens in Small Spaces

The question I am asked most often is about creating herbal tea gardens in pots, on decks, on kitchen windowsills, and so on. Like so many of us, I have limited space around my little home, and growing herbs indoors is the obvious way to go, particularly since many herbs are not exceptionally large and grow happily in pots.

Unfortunately, it's also possible to become a herb killer of note (yes, I am talking about myself here) if some simple and basic rules aren't followed. Herbs are different from many of the other indoor plants we may be familiar with, but as long as one follows a few basic guidelines, it should be possible to have a decent range of herbs for tea growing in your kitchen or on your deck for most of the year (depending on your weather zone, of course).

To avoid problems with your herbal tea plants, the first thing you need to consider is the light available in your kitchen or growing area (or lack thereof). Direct light is needed by most herbs if they are to survive and thrive; this is partly because many of the most popular herbs come from the hot and bright Mediterranean regions of the world. Place your herb pots in areas or on windowsills where they will get the maximum amount of light—in general this is south-facing. Cold is also a factor, and the reality is that some herbs will probably not survive cold and dark winters, even indoors. (Basil and cilantro are two such herbs, as they need lots of warmth and direct, bright sunlight.) If your weather has turned cold, move the pots away from the windows at night, and keep them in the warmer places of your house. You could also move the pots outside during the day into a sheltered patch of sunshine.

Other problems arise from both underwatering (for moisture-loving herbs like basil) and overwatering (for the more hardy types like rosemary). In general, though, herbs don't like to have wet feet, as ultimately this can lead to root rot. This problem can be partly resolved by ensuring your pots and containers have plenty of drainage by layering the bottom of the pot with small pebbles and stones. Also, don't use garden soil for herbs in containers—they need light well-draining soil, preferably a mixture of potting soil, peat/coir, and perlite.

Herbs can be grown together in window boxes or larger containers and look very pretty, but not all make happy

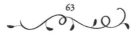

companions! Rosemary and thyme, for example, grow well together, but mint should always be given its own space. (Quite apart from the fact that it tends to take over everything!) Also remember that herbs grow more slowly indoors, so only harvest limited amounts of the plant at any one time, thus giving it time to bounce back and remain healthy.

Herbs can also be grown in hanging baskets on decks and patios, which looks very charming, but position is very important if you are going to grow herbs in these types of containers. Herbs do not like full sun all day or being exposed to lots of wind, so be aware of this when positioning your hanging baskets; also, don't overcrowd the baskets. Herbs generally grow fast, and if too cramped they will not flourish but start to lose their leaves and droop. They also benefit from being picked regularly, so make sure that's possible with your hanging baskets. Some herbs that work well in hanging baskets are creeping thymes, catmint, marjoram, some of the mint family, and prostrate (creeping) rosemary. Lots of flowers grow well in hanging baskets, such as nasturtiums and wild pansies (heartsease).

As a starter plan for an indoor herb tea garden—and depending on your environmental conditions and the size of your container—the following herbs are all potentially suitable: mint, rosemary, thyme, oregano, basil, lemon balm, parsley, cilantro, and sage.

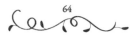

PART 3
Tea Witch
Enchantments

Never waste any amount of time doing anything important when there is a sunset outside that you should be sitting under!

C. JoyBell C.

9

Astrological Teas

The position of the sun at the time of our birth is indicative of our general personality traits. We can use our star signs as heavenly signposts to guide our path through life.

It is a little simplistic to say that "one size fits all" when it comes to astrological signs, as we are all highly complex beings, in addition to the fact that we all have our own life experiences that shape us for good or ill, but in general there are certain personality traits and ways of being that are particular to each sign. Some of these are positive; some have more negative connotations (ask me: I am a Scorpio and have heard quite a few strange stories about this particular sign).

However, it's not often realized that because each sign has particular herbs, flowers, and plants linked to it, we can

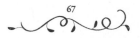

also use this information as part of our herbal tea journey by creating specific tea blends and mixtures for each of the signs. The ideas given below are just a brief starting point: you will probably find inspiration for making your own uniquely healing and helpful blends as you explore this further. These sun/moon sign tea blends make a special and unique gift, particularly on the birthday of the person involved. Why not plan a special astrological tea party for them on their special day?

Aries Often impulsive and quick to make decisions, Arians can make natural leaders and have the desire to carve their own independent path through life, creating new challenges and opportunities. On the darker side, Aries can battle to show or understand emotions and are sometimes insensitive to the needs of others. Plants that are linked to Aries include clove, fennel, rosemary, juniper, dandelion, and peppermint.

Taurus A generally happy-go-lucky sign, Taurus appreciates the finer things in life and is sensual by nature. However, Taurus can find change difficult and prefer to stick with rituals they know and understand. A key lesson for this sign is learning to be flexible and flow with life and its inevitable changes. Plants for Taurus include rose, thyme, catnip, vanilla, apple, violet, and hibiscus.

Gemini   People born under this sign are mentally agile and have lots of ideas, even if sometimes they battle to follow through on them. Fairly prone to stress and tension, they tend to move on quickly when situations (or other people) become uncomfortable for them and thus often miss opportunities for personal growth and understanding. Enjoying mental stimulation and the lighter side of life, they also need to learn the value of silence and of taking the time to put ideas into concrete action. Tea blends that could be useful for Gemini include bergamot, lavender, lemongrass, mint, parsley, hawthorn, and dill.

Cancer   A generally sensitive, caring, and emotional sign with well-developed intuition and psychic abilities. Cancers are the carers of the world, often taking on and trying to solve other people's problems instead of allowing them to take responsibility for themselves. Because of these traits, Cancers are both loving and

also possessive, with a tendency to moodiness and "poor me" syndrome. Learning to balance emotions is an important goal for this sign, and plants that are linked with this include jasmine, rose, lemon balm, eucalyptus, and lemon.

Leo Rather like their namesake, Leos are proud and strong, sometimes a little flamboyant, and always willing to stick their necks out. Born extroverts, they are drawn to creative activities of all kinds but have to guard against becoming egotistical or self-centred. However, they are great at inspiring others and are also very romantic and loving at heart. Spicy, warm notes are typical of Leo herbs and plants such as cinnamon, nutmeg, orange, marigold, St. John's wort, rosemary, and juniper.

Virgo People born in this sign are practical and methodical, with a need to have everything in its place. However, this can make them a little critical or judgemental of others who don't share their meticulous nature, so flexibility is an important lesson for them. On the positive side, they are also the peacemakers and diplomats of the star signs, and generally make loving and reliable partners and parents—although sometimes they need to learn to loosen up a little! Plants suitable for Virgo include mint, thyme, bergamot, lavender, fennel, and vervain.

Libra   Librans are charming, likeable, and generally sensitive to the feelings of others, which can lead to them being taken advantage of on an emotional level. Because they love beauty in all things, they are naturally creative and enjoy making their surroundings as attractive as possible. Loving partners in relationships, they try to avoid disharmony at home, as this can lead to physical and stress-related health issues. Libra plants include catnip, marjoram, ashwagandha, nettle, yarrow, mugwort, rooibos, thyme, and spearmint.

Scorpio   The intuitive, deep sign known for keeping secrets and, unfortunately, sometimes harboring grudges. Scorpios don't forgive easily, either others or what they perceive as their own failures, and this can lead to issues like addiction, negativity, and depression. However, Scorpios are extremely talented and known for their gifts in healing work of all kinds. Above all, people

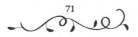

born under this sign need to learn to forgive and move on, to let go of what is past and embrace a brighter future. Plants for Scorpio include basil, cumin, ginger, hops, geranium, hibiscus, and borage.

Sagittarius Gregarious, witty, individualistic, and funny, people born under this sign are talented and very able in whatever they choose to do but can also lack sensitivity towards the needs and rights of others around them. Sagittarians need to be stimulated mentally or they become restless and sometimes a little self-destructive. Loving partners and parents, they need their surroundings to be happy and optimistic ones, otherwise they tend to move on, looking for more positive landscapes and outcomes. Tea blends for this sign can include anise, fennel, dandelion, star anise, honeysuckle, and nutmeg.

Capricorn Hardworking and driven to succeed, sometimes at the cost of personal relationships, Capricorns will possibly make a lot of money and become famous, but the price can be high, and they often become emotionally detached and physically burnt out. This sign benefits from learning to laugh, lighten up, be spontaneous, live in the moment, and accept that emotional success is vitally necessary for a balanced and joyful life. Capricorn plants include lemon thyme, skullcap, California poppy, chamomile, and vervain.

Aquarius Original and creative thinkers, Aquarians are independent and outspoken; they love freedom and are often inspired to improve the world around them. Drawn to the mysterious and supernatural, people of this sign are deep and sometimes secretive, which can make them something of an enigma to those around them. They generally need to find a balance between ideas and action and ground themselves so that they don't suffer from nervous tension or confusion. Plants linked to this sign include fennel, lavender, pine, mint, lemongrass, parsley, and hops.

Pisces A sensitive, kind, and compassionate sign, Pisceans are generally deeply spiritual and sensitive to all kinds of mysteries and undercurrents. They are creative, although they often lack true confidence in their own innate creativity. They don't like conflict and sometimes

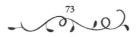

will do anything to keep the peace, even if this means procrastinating or telling a few mistruths! However, they make loving and loyal partners as long as they are understood and their deep emotional commitment is not abused in any way. Plants for this sign include lemon balm, bergamot, rose, sage, passionflower, chamomile, willow, and linden.

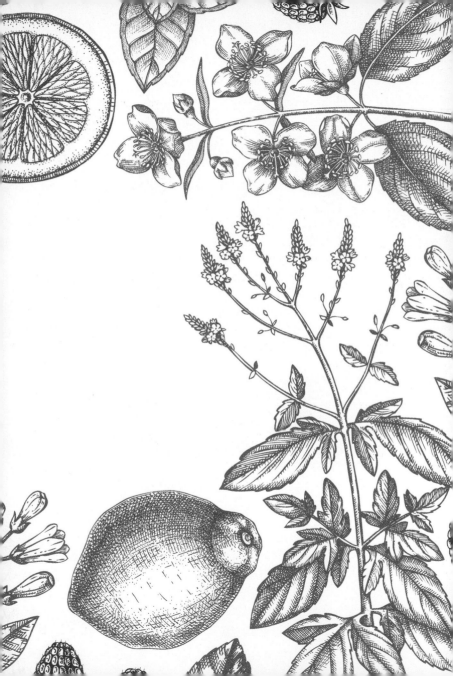

A Proper Tea is much nicer
than a Very Nearly Tea, which is
one you forget about afterwards.

A. A. Milne

10

Making Herbal Tea Syrups

*A*lthough in general I prefer to use limited quantities of sugar in tea, there is a place for herbal tea syrups, especially in the making of iced tea. They can also be stored and used for adding to warming winter tea infusions, as sugar is a natural preservative. The syrups should be kept in small glass jars or bottles with tight lids, preferably in the refrigerator, for no more than a month or two.

Fresh Herb Syrup

Combine ½ cup each water and sugar in a small saucepan and add a pinch of salt. You can also add ½ teaspoon vanilla extract, but that's optional. Bring the syrup to boil and then add 4 sprigs of fresh herbs such as mint, thyme, basil, rosemary, or lemon verbena. Cover the pan and

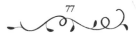

simmer very gently for 20–25 minutes. Strain, cool, and then pour the syrup into a suitable bottle or jar.

Spice Syrups

These are particularly good in wintertime teas! Another alternative is to add a tea bag or two to the syrup—this can be black tea (such as Earl Grey or rooibos) or a flower tea (such as jasmine or green tea). I also use both herb and spice syrups to add a little extra flavor to baked goods or desserts by drizzling a little syrup over them before serving.

Cardamom Syrup

One of the most delightful spices, and deliciously warming, too! Toast a few cardamom pods lightly in a frying pan (or purchase already crushed seeds), then crush them in a mortar and pestle. (You can add a few vanilla seeds too for extra flavor.) Combine ¼ cup brown sugar with 1 cup water and simmer over a low heat until the sugar has dissolved. Add the crushed cardamom and continue to cook over a low heat for 10–15 minutes. Remove from the heat, cool, and strain thoroughly before storing in small glass bottles or jars.

Ginger and Spice Tea Syrup

This particular recipe is very warming and packed with powerful healing properties. You can stir a spoonful into cups of herbal or black tea or simply add it to boiling water and drink it as-is. Please only use fresh ginger—for some reason it doesn't work as well with ground ginger.

In a saucepan, combine 1 cup water, ½ cup sugar, and 2 tablespoons finely chopped fresh ginger root. Bring to a low simmer, then add 2 cinnamon sticks, a few cloves, and a teaspoon of nutmeg. Cook slowly for 10 minutes or until the syrup is slightly thickened, then remove from the heat and cool. Strain the syrup into a small glass jar and keep in a cool, dark place. It should be used within 2 to 3 weeks.

MAKES ABOUT 1¼ CUPS SYRUP

Close your eyes and follow
your breath to the still place
that leads to the invisible
path that leads you home.

St. Teresa of Avila

11

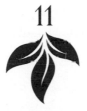

Flower Essences

*A*s I am a trained flower essence therapist and work with them on many levels, I am often asked if they can be included in teatime rituals or added to the teas we drink. The answer to that is yes, happily, in all but a few limited cases. As we green witches know, flower essences are a true gift from the flower spirits and Mother Earth herself, bringing the sacred and healing vibrations of each plant within our reach in a simple and safe way.

Adding a few drops of essence to your cup of tea is a delightful way of accessing these gifts and magic every day; however, I would suggest that you choose your tea with care and insight. Very strong or dark teas can remove the soft, subtle vibrations of many essences, so a light green tea is often the better choice. Similarly, boiling hot water

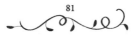

is not conducive to maintaining the gentle magic of the essences, so it's better to only add them when the tea has cooled off somewhat. Obviously, they are ideally suited to adding to iced teas and other chilled drinks and can make a seemingly ordinary beverage something truly effective and spiritual.

You can use purchased flower essences for tea purposes. There are a number of amazing ones on the market, starting with the classic range by Dr. Edward Bach, who first made flower essences known in Western countries. However, making your own flower essences is an easy and magical process, for each of us will be instinctively drawn to flowers or plants that call to our own personal energies. Perhaps you will find these flowers in your own garden, on a walk in the country, or even at the local farmers market. When making essences you don't need to worry if a plant is edible or even poisonous since flower essences do not carry traces of the original plant. This gives you some more options, as obviously some herbs and flowers are toxic when ingested as teas or infusions. Having said that, although some herbalists do make essences with toxic plants such as foxglove or datura, I prefer to err on the side of caution and stick to plants I know to be safe.

The first step is, obviously, to choose flowers or plants that you feel a connection with, that speak to your soul and spirit on some deep level. On a clear sunny day (this is very important), fill a large glass bowl with spring water and place it in full sunshine. Generally you need a few handfuls of flowers or plant material, which should be gathered gently into a flat basket so as to handle them as little as possible; use small scissors or plant shears to cut them gently and drop them into the basket. Then float the plants on the surface of the water and leave in full sun for at least two hours. After this time you can remove the plants, using a twig or something similar to scoop them out. Again, you want to handle them as little as possible, so that you don't transfer too much of your own energy into the liquid.

Scatter the plant material at the base of a tree while giving thanks to Mother Earth for her beautiful gifts so freely shared with us. Then pour the water into a large sterilized dark glass bottle until it is half full. Fill the bottle up to the top with brandy or vodka. You have now created the mother essence. Label and date this bottle. To create flower essence bottles for everyday use, take 4–7 drops of the mother essence and put them into small 1-ounce dark glass dropper bottles. Fill with your chosen alcohol, label, and date. To use the flower essences, add a few drops to a glass of spring water, a cup of warm tea, or directly under the tongue. Flower essences can also be added to a tub of warm

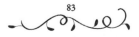

bath water. Moon essences are basically made in the same way but created under the light of a full moon.

Here is a very short list of flowers you may choose to use for making essences and their magical correspondences. I have not included flowers or other plants widely used for making teas and infusions.

Camellia   being authentic, learning true wisdom

Carnation   healing the heart, love, true passion

Chrysanthemum   protection, longevity

Daisy   natural healing, innocence, relief from stress and anxiety

Forget-Me-Not   clarifying the mind, memory, intention

Geranium (all varieties)   magical protection, good health, healing on all levels

Iris   wisdom, finding our inner truth, being more creative

Lilac   balancing our inner beings, stepping into other realms and possibilities

Lily   divine energies, protection, finding harmony in our lives

Magnolia   ancient goddess wisdom and
remembering our personal power

Morning Glory   awakening to the gift that is our
lives, intuition, and happiness

Pansy   finding beauty in our own being, opening
up to divine inspiration, clarity

Snapdragon   strong protection against harmful
forces, speaking our truth

Sunflower   health, vitality, finding new happiness
and meaning

Tulip   beauty, gratitude, strengthening and healing
the heart

Water Lily   balancing emotions, allowing inner
wisdom to flow

Wisteria   coping with ageing, healing grief, seeing
the blessings in our lives

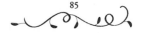

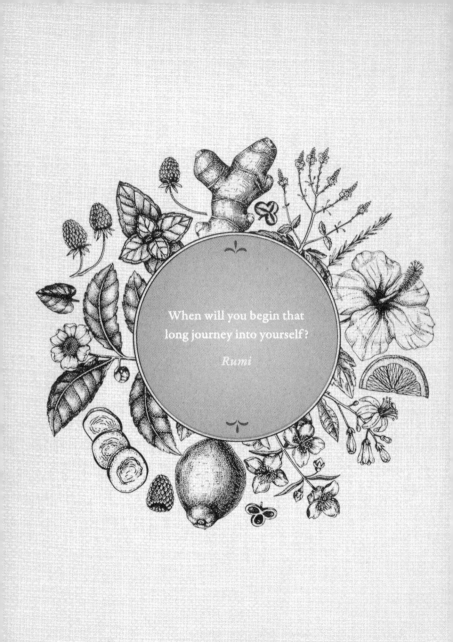

When will you begin that
long journey into yourself?

Rumi

12

Tea Blends for Chakra Wisdom & Healing

The chakras are an ancient Sanskrit system of describing and defining different energy centres in the body. These seven centres are not only related to physical aspects such as organs and glands, but also emotional states of being. If our chakras are blocked in some way—through illness, perhaps, or emotional issues— energy becomes blocked and we experience ill health and psychological difficulties. Herbs, spices, and other plants are often indicated for use with the different chakras, and in my first book, *Enchanted Herbal*, I offered some ideas for creating essential oil blends that would be supportive and healing of our seven chakras.

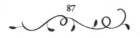

Teas, too, can be used for this, and below you will find a list of the seven chakras, their colors and energy fields they represent, and some ideas for teas suitable for each.

Base Chakra Located at the bottom of the spine. Red. The energies of abundance, inner strength, stability, and being grounded. Teas could include elderflower, sage, thyme, peppermint, and dandelion.

Sacral Chakra Located in the lower abdomen. Orange. Sexuality and love of life in all its facets, accepting pleasure and sensuality. Teas to support these energies include hibiscus, raspberry leaf, rose, jasmine, and calendula.

Solar Plexus Chakra Located in the upper abdomen. Yellow. Balance and focus, greater self-esteem and sense of purpose, vitality. Possible herbal teas are lemon balm, peppermint, rosemary, ginger, fennel, and cinnamon.

Heart Chakra Located in the heart and lungs. Green. Giving and receiving love on all levels, balanced and healthy relationships, self-acceptance and compassion. Rose, oatstraw, geranium, jasmine, linden, and hawthorn are all possible teas to support this chakra.

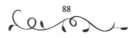

Throat Chakra   Located in the throat and thyroid gland. Light blue. Clarity, creativity, and being able to communicate our truth with honesty. Teas to support this include chamomile, sage, peppermint, rosemary, and eucalyptus.

Brow Chakra   Located in the area between and above the eyes. Dark blue or indigo. Perception and insight, imagination, and the achievement of true purpose. Consider trying teas made with lemon, spearmint, hops, juniper, or mugwort.

Crown Chakra   Located at the very top of the head. White or light purple. Our highest and most sacred self, the wisdom that leads to true enlightenment and inner peace. Teas for this chakra include rose, elderflower, lemon balm, bergamot, lavender, and sage.

These are just some general suggestions; obviously you may find other herbs or plants that work particularly well for you as regards the individual chakras.

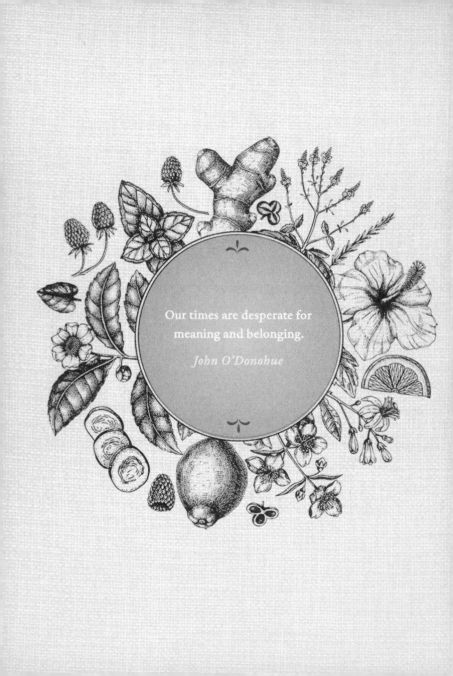

Our times are desperate for
meaning and belonging.

John O'Donohue

13

The Oracle of the Leaves

ea leaf reading, referred to as tasseomancy or tasseography, is one of the most ancient forms of divination and looking into the future; it's probably been around as long as the drinking of tea itself, at least 5,000 years! However, it first became really popular in the West during Victorian times in Great Britain, when it was a fashionable trend among the upper classes to employ Romany fortunetellers to read tea leaves and predict the future. Today this ancient art continues to live on, and green witches from all countries and belief systems use it as a way of accessing wisdom and natural intuitive forces.

While I certainly don't pretend to be an expert on this subject (and there are a number of excellent books available should you want to pursue this in greater depth), here are just a few short ideas to get you started.

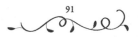

Tea leaf reading can be done with either green or black tea leaves, which tend to be easier to read in the cup. While herbal teas (made with dried leaves) can be used, if the tea includes spices or other large pieces of plant material, they will affect the outcome of the reading or make it impossible to see the images. Do not be tempted to open a tea bag (herbal or otherwise) and use it for this purpose; the tea in bags is often somewhat pulverized and will simply form clumps.

Before preparing your tea, take a few moments to sit quietly and reflect on what it is you are hoping to gain from this reading. Questions you might like to ask yourself (or anyone else you are doing the reading for) include the following:

- How am I feeling today in body and spirit?

- What do I need to do today for my own best interests?

- Are my energies in a good place?

- Are there specific things I need to change in my life right now?

- What dreams and goals do I have at this moment?

- How can I move in the direction of my dreams?

- What am I hoping for in the future?

This is a wonderful activity for teas that celebrate soul, spirit, and divination on any level, such as teas for Samhain, Halloween, and other seasonal changes. I would also suggest using it at the Spirits and Memories Tea in part 4.

Reading the Leaves

When you have made the tea, which in this case obviously must be made with loose leaves, drink it slowly and reverently until there are just a few teaspoons of cool tea in the bottom of the cup. Use a plain, light-colored china cup for this ritual, if possible; mugs are not generally suitable because of their straight sides.

Gently swirl the cup three times: clockwise, counterclockwise, and then clockwise again. Set the cup down on a firm surface, close your eyes, and breathe deeply three times. Then look into the cup, allowing yourself to see any shapes or other images that may have formed within the tea leaves. If there are none discernible, add a few spoons of cooled boiled water and swirl the cup again.

This does actually take some practice, and for the first few times you may think all you are seeing is an indistinct lump of tea leaves, but give it time and certain definite images will start to become apparent.

The position of the tea leaves within the cup is also important: if they are near the top of the cup, they signify

THE ORACLE OF THE LEAVES

things and events happening in the present, your current situation, or any issues you may be having. These situations may require your immediate attention and need to be dealt with soon.

Tea leaves forming patterns down the sides of the cup are indicative of things to come in the relatively near future: what may change in your life or issues that need to be addressed going forward—for example, in a difficult relationship or financial problems. You can take time to reflect on these and plan accordingly. The tea leaves at the very bottom of the cup are a portent of longer-term events and changes in your life—perhaps travelling, meeting someone new, or other significant shifts in your path forward. They are something to look forward to and work towards in the long term but not necessarily something that requires your immediate focus and action.

There are many different ways of interpreting the images or symbols you may see within the tea leaves. A search online or in books will undoubtedly give you much more insight into this ancient skill, but here is a short list of some of the more commonly found symbols and their generally accepted meaning:

Birds   freedom, travel

Fish   good luck

Butterfly   faith, eternal secrets

Dog   friendship

Heart   new love, strengthening existing bonds
of affection

Sun   success and happiness

Knife or sword   danger, awareness of possible
pitfalls and negative energies

Cross   blocked energy, doubts

Anchor   faith, being grounded

Moon and stars   following the light, trusting in
the mystery of life

House   making changes

Cat   hidden secrets

Mountains   obstacles and blockages to be faced,
new beginnings

Angel   a very positive symbol, a sign of being
supported and protected

Boat   travel, making changes in your life,
moving on

Candle   peace, spiritual enlightenment

Cup or chalice   positive sacrifices, settling emotions, finding a way back to peace

Feathers   spiritual growth and awareness; a need for quiet, introspective time

Spirals   connection to the divine; new enlightenment in any area of life

Star   finding new hope, faith, and purpose; wishes that are coming true

PART 4

*Teas for Every
Day, Season
&
Celebration*

There are only two ways to live your life. One is as though nothing is a miracle. The other is as though everything is a miracle.

Albert Einstein

14

Tea at Sunrise

Sunrise—the beginning of a new day, with all its as-yet-unknown gifts and promise (and yes, sometimes challenges too!). It's long been known that the early hours of the morning, just before and after sunrise, are the time when we are at our most open and receptive to creativity, inspiration, and magic, for we have not yet had the chance to become bogged down in the demands and stresses of the day.

I love getting up as the sky starts to lighten and sitting out on my deck, if the weather permits, with that first cup of tea, listening to the happy sounds of the birds waking up and the wind off the sea rustling the leaves of the trees around my little house. I have come to cherish this particular morning tea ritual and try to enjoy it at least a few times a week.

Teatime at sunrise? It might seem a little strange for those of us who think teatime has a more strictly defined time frame, generally mid morning or late afternoon. But I personally believe the magic of tea is something we could and should enjoy at any time of the day and in any place—which is one of the reasons I wrote this little book!

Of course, teatime at sunrise is probably more likely than most to be a solitary affair, but that is not necessarily a negative thing. It gives us a chance to reflect, quietly and in silence, about the day ahead and what we hope to bring to it on every level. This quiet time can help us settle our thoughts, reframe any anxieties we may have, and clarify our goals. For this reason, writing or drawing in a journal is particularly helpful at this time and encourages us to begin the day on a positive note. If you are familiar with Julia Cameron's wonderful book *The Artist's Way*, you will remember the "morning pages" exercise she endorses, which suggests that a few pages of free writing helps set the tone for a truly creative and healthy day.

Whether you have a solitary tea at sunrise or share it with others, there are several ways in which you can make it especially meaningful.

For starters, if you are like me and prefer a calm and non-stressful start to the morning, it's a good idea to have a morning tea tray ready. Mine is very simple: just a small bamboo tray that holds a pretty teacup, a few tea bags, and a tiny jar of honey, and always a little extra touch—perhaps a fresh flower or sprig of rosemary and a small book of affirmations to read.

I prepare the tea tray in the late evening, cover it with a light cloth, and leave it in a corner of my kitchen; then, in the morning, all I have to do is fill up and boil the kettle to start my simple tea ceremony. If it's winter and still dark or the weather is grey and gloomy, I use a few candles to bring the colors of sunrise into my home—yellow, gold, and soft pink are my favorites. A little gentle incense is also appropriate and helps focus the mind in a peaceful way. I love using lavender, geranium, or rose as they create such a beautiful and tranquil start to the day.

As an additional note: you might want to choose a fairly strong and robust tea like English breakfast, which gives a little kick-start to the day! However, if you would prefer something lighter and lower in caffeine, Earl Grey with a slice of lemon works well too. Actually, any herbal tea from the mint or citrus family is a good choice for an early morning cup, and a sprig of rosemary in your tea will ensure bright and clear thinking as you move into your day.

Sunrise is happening every day. It's a beautiful gift from the earth and heavens just waiting for us. All we have to do is open our eyes. The beauty is there, freely given.

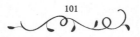

This is a simple sunrise ritual I try to do before sitting down with my tea and often something small and delicious to eat. Stand facing the east (or light an appropriate candle if need be) and quietly say the following words:

The day we have been given is here. We are blessed and grateful. Whatever this day holds, we accept its gifts and promise. Every day we are reminded of life and the magic of this earth; may we always honor and cherish this simple blessing. And so it is!

Bright New Day Tea Blend

This is a lovely, fresh, and energising tea blend, full of bright flavor and color; use it to make a beautiful start to your day and allow it to infuse you with new hope, focus, and creative ideas.

Use 1–2 teaspoons of the mix in a cup of just-boiled water, infuse for 10 minutes, strain, and add honey, maple syrup, or stevia to sweeten as required. This tea calls for dried orange zest, but if you don't have any on hand, you can use a little very finely grated fresh orange zest instead.

Combine ½ cup dried peppermint leaves, ¼ cup dried marigold petals, 2 stalks of very finely chopped dried lemongrass, 2 teaspoons dried orange zest, and 1 teaspoon ground ginger in a small bowl, and mix together well.

Transfer to a suitable airtight jar or tin for storage. The tea should keep its freshness and flavor for a couple of months if stored in a dark and cool spot.

Mood Lifter Tea

Sometimes, despite our best intentions, we wake in the morning feeling anxious and stressed, particularly if we know that particular day will hold its own set of challenges. On such days it can be very tempting to just pull the covers over our head and not get up at all!

The gentle ingredients contained in this tea blend will help lift our mood and enable us to face the new day with greater equanimity and a positive outlook. Please note that St. John's wort is a powerful herb and should be used with caution, especially if you are already taking medication for anxiety and depression; consult your healthcare professional first.

Place one chamomile tea bag in your mug, then add 1 teaspoon each dried St. John's wort leaves, peppermint, marjoram, and a pinch of ground cinnamon. Pour one cup of just-boiled water over the herbs, steep for 10 minutes, then strain and drink slowly and mindfully, breathing in the uplifting qualities of the herbs and spices.

Esther's Morning Tea

Esther, a beautiful red-haired friend of mine, swears by this tea blend to start the morning on a fresh and healing note. She generally makes it the evening before and serves it chilled on summer mornings, but I imagine it would also be delightful served warm when the weather is chilly! The rooibos tea is such a favorite for its antioxidant and healing properties, and it works really well with the floral and lemon flavors of the herbs.

To make 4 cups of tea, make a pot of rooibos tea with 4 cups of just-boiled water and 3–4 rooibos tea bags. Stir in 3–4 crushed rose geranium leaves, a few lemon verbena leaves, and 1 tablespoon dried lavender blossoms. Allow to steep for 15 minutes, then strain and refrigerate until serving time. It's nice with ice on a sultry summer morning.

Lavender-Basil Tea

This is a simple and fresh way to start the morning, leaving behind the problems of the previous day and enjoying being in the moment. It's also a lovely tea for all kinds of parties since almost everyone enjoys it.

Simply place ½ cup fresh basil leaves (or 2 tablespoons dried) in a teapot together with 2 teaspoons fresh lavender leaves/flowers (or 1 teaspoon dried) and 3–4 cups just-boiled water. Allow to steep for 10–15 minutes, then pour through a strainer into the teacups. This tea can be sweetened with a little floral honey if you like, but try it unsweetened first to really appreciate the intense green and floral aroma and taste!

Red (Rooibos) Cappucino

For those of us who have been addicted to our early morning cup of joe, this makes a far more healthful substitute, without caffeine and packed with healthy antioxidants! You simply brew a strong cup of rooibos tea (sweetened or not, as you prefer) and then top with steamed milk that you have beaten up to a light froth (I use a small hand whisk for this). You can use either dairy milk or an alternative such as almond or soya milk. Pile the milk on top of the tea and then sprinkle with a little finely ground cinnamon or nutmeg.

Earl Grey Tea Bread

I know I am not alone when I say that Earl Grey is one of my favorite teas, with its delicate, refreshing, and uplifting taste and fragrance, warmed with the delicacy of bergamot. Earl Grey tea also works wonderfully well when used in recipes, especially for baked goods! This tea bread recipe adds the flavor of oranges, dates, and golden raisins for a delicious and healthful treat, which can be served on its

own or sliced and buttered (which is how my mom always did it, but then she believed that butter simply made everything taste better). This bread just seems perfect to start the day; it has a vitality and positive vibe that is a good note on which to begin.

Preheat oven to 325°F.

Grease and line a medium bread pan.

3 Earl Grey tea bags

1¼ cups boiling water

4 ounces pitted dates, chopped

¾ cup golden raisins

1 cup light brown sugar

1 stick butter

1 teaspoon baking soda

2 cups flour

½ teaspoon salt

1 teaspoon ground cinnamon

2 eggs, beaten

1 tablespoon orange zest

Place the tea bags in a glass jug and pour the boiling water over them. Steep for 10 minutes, then remove the tea bags. Combine the tea, dates, raisins, sugar, and butter in a saucepan and simmer very gently for 10 minutes or until the sugar has dissolved and the butter is melted. Stir in the baking soda, then remove from the heat and cool for 15 minutes.

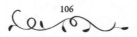

In a large bowl, sift together the flour, salt, and cinnamon, then stir in the cooled fruit mixture, the eggs, and the orange zest. Beat to make a thick batter, then pour it into the prepared pan and bake for 1¼ hours or until the loaf is golden brown and it tests done. Cool briefly in the pan before turning out onto a wire rack. This loaf can be kept, wrapped, for up to 4 days.

Morning Glory Muffins

Moist and delicious, these are a simple early morning treat that can replace breakfast. All the fruit and nuts make them seem remarkably healthy, and the cinnamon adds a warming and healing note. You can also mix the batter the night before and leave it in a covered bowl in the refrigerator overnight before baking up the muffins in the morning. I like to make them mini sized but regular works well, too.

Preheat oven to 350°F.

Grease a 12-cup (or 24-cup mini) muffin pan well.

2 cups flour

2 teaspoons baking powder

1 teaspoon ground cinnamon

½ teaspoon salt

½ cup unsweetened shredded coconut

2 eggs

½ cup sugar

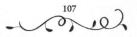

½ cup vegetable oil

1 teaspoon vanilla extract

1 apple, peeled and grated

1 carrot, peeled and grated

½ cup seedless raisins

½ cup chopped pecans (optional)

Sift the flour, baking powder, cinnamon, salt, and coconut together in a large bowl. In another bowl, beat the eggs, sugar, oil, and vanilla together until thick and creamy. Add to the flour mixture together with the apple, carrot, raisins, and pecans, and beat quickly—the mixture should be thick and lumpy; don't overmix.

Fill the prepared muffin tins ¾ full with the batter and bake for 20–25 minutes until risen and golden brown. Cool in the pans for 5 minutes before turning out onto a wire rack. The muffins will keep in an airtight container for a few days.

Ginger-Almond Butter Cookies

These little cookies, full of bright and positive energy, make the ideal accompaniment to your first cup of tea in the morning. An added benefit is that they can be made in advance and stored in the refrigerator or freezer so in the morning all you have to do is slice and bake for fresh cookies. If you would like to increase the ginger factor, you can add a tablespoon of very finely grated fresh ginger or finely chopped crystallized ginger to the mixture. The almonds add another magical note but can be excluded if there are allergy issues.

Preheat oven to 300°F.

Grease a large cookie sheet well.

> **2 sticks unsalted butter, softened**
> **⅔ cup light brown sugar**
> **1 teaspoon vanilla extract**
> **2 cups cake flour**
> **1 tablespoon ground ginger**
> **½ teaspoon baking powder**
> **¼ teaspoon salt**
> **½ teaspoon ground cardamom**
> **1 tablespoon grated fresh ginger**
> **¼ cup flaked almonds**

In a large bowl cream the butter, sugar, and vanilla together until the mixture is light and fluffy. In another bowl sift together the flour, ginger, baking powder, salt, and cardamom, then add this to the butter mixture to form a soft dough. Stir in the ginger if you are using it. Chill the dough for 30 minutes, then shape it into two or more logs, 1½ inches in diameter. Roll the logs up in baking paper and keep in the fridge for up to a week or in the freezer for up to a month.

When you want to bake the cookies, allow a roll to warm up for 10 minutes, then use a very sharp knife to cut cookies about ¼-inch thick. Arrange on a cookie sheet and sprinkle a few flaked almonds on each cookie. Bake for 10–15 minutes or until the cookies are a very light golden brown. Cool on a wire rack. These cookies can be stored in an airtight container for a week.

MAKES ABOUT 48 COOKIES

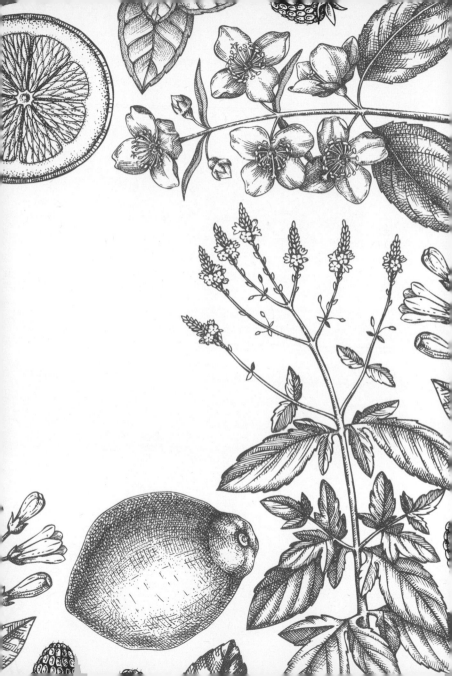

Home wasn't ... a place, but a moment, and then another, building on each other like bricks to create a solid shelter that you take with you for your entire life, wherever you may go.

Sarah Dessen

15

Kitchen Table Teas

In my mother's kitchen she had a little hand-painted sign; bright and colorful, very '70s in style, it hung there as long as I can remember. "Wherever I serve my guests, it seems they like my kitchen best." My teenage self thought that was both trite and old-fashioned, and I am sure I told my mom that several times. Wisely, she ignored me, because she knew the truth; a truth that it took me a little longer to discover in its simple wisdom. Not for nothing is the kitchen known as the heart of the home, and, more importantly, it is the center of the wisdom, magic, and grace we can create very simply every day. Kitchen witchery, indeed.

As I said in the introduction, I grew up with tea as part and parcel of everyday life—not only the special tea parties that were a feature of birthday and other milestone

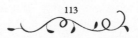

events, but also the everyday tea that usually happened around 4 o'clock in the afternoon. The electric kettle would be switched on and the teapot and blue-and-white Noritake teacups arranged on the kitchen table. Sometimes there would be cake from the candy-striped tin at the top of the cupboard, but more often there would be rusks or simple butter cookies. This quiet time, either just my mom and me or with any people who happened to be visiting, was just a part of our day's daily pattern.

It was only as I grew older that I learned a little more about why this ritual was so important to my mother. She had been born in Cape Town just before the start of the second world war; her family, which also consisted of her mother, father, and older brother, did not have an easy time of it financially and often lived, as my mom used to put it, from hand to mouth. After the end of the war, when she was seven, the family lost their little home and had to rent an apartment in a boarding house, a small and cramped space where the two children had to sleep on the covered porch. Yet, as my mom told me, there was always a sense of abundance and joy in her home, and every afternoon the kettle would be boiled and tea poured and drunk in an atmosphere of grace and hope. They had very little, but they made sure they enjoyed and savored the moment, grateful for the companionship and love they shared.

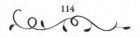

And I believe this is the early lesson my mother never forgot, and one which she passed on to me: share what you have, even if it's very simple. Be grateful for the moment. Make every day something to celebrate, no matter what your situation. Remember how blessed we are, especially in those we love and those who love us. It's all about connection, and I believe that is what kitchen table teas mean, simple and unpretentious though they may be.

Sitting around the table we can let go of the need to be anything other than who we are. We can truly share our hearts and selves. I have had many of my most open and honest—even if sometimes painful—conversations at the kitchen table, sipping tea and just being present in that moment.

So, kitchen table teas are simple and abundant at the same time. They don't need fancy cups or table decorations, although a jug of wildflowers and herbs is always welcome; what they need is the warmth of connection and friendship and the joy of being together in moments that are both memorable and precious.

Tea, of course, represents all of the earth's elements: air, water, earth, and fire, and a simple grace reflecting this is a lovely way to begin or conclude a kitchen table tea. Gather around the table, boil the water, and prepare the tea. Everyone present should lift their cup or mug and say:

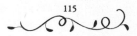

*Air, water, earth, fire … all these gifts of
our world are here. But more than that
are the unseen gifts, the blessings we share
of love, of friendship, of community. May
this tea and this time always remind us
of the grace and gifts we celebrate and
share in this quiet and sacred hour.*

Everyday Health Tea

This rooibos-based tea blend is based on one from the
book *Tea* by the late Margaret Roberts, the doyenne of
South African herb writers. Even those of us who aren't
that keen on the flavor of rooibos, like me, find this tea palatable and refreshing. It makes a good kitchen table tea as
it is simple, cleansing, and good for us on many levels both
physical and emotional.

This recipe makes one cup but can easily be increased to
serve as many as you need. Place 1 rooibos tea bag in the
cup and add a thin slice of lemon, 2 very thin slices of fresh
ginger, 3 cloves, and a few fresh lemon balm or spearmint
leaves. Pour a cup of just-boiled water over the ingredients and allow to steep for 5–10 minutes. Strain and serve
sweetened with honey. This tea can also be served cold over
some crushed ice.

"Talking It Over" Tea Blend

One of the most important things we do is communicate with each other, but sometimes various factors make that difficult; we put off having certain conversations for a number of different reasons and ultimately end up feeling disconnected, uncomfortable, and stressed. Sitting around the kitchen table is one of the most nonthreatening and pleasant ways to have conversations of any kind, and this simple, spicy tea blend contains the necessary ingredients to support that—caraway seeds, lemon for clarity of thought, and cinnamon and thyme for courage and strength.

In a small bowl combine 1 teaspoon caraway seeds, a thin slice of fresh lemon, ½ a cinnamon stick (crushed), and 1 teaspoon dried thyme (or 1 tablespoon fresh thyme leaves). Pour 1 cup of just-boiled water over the herbs and steep for 10 minutes. Strain and serve warm; a little honey and a drop of vanilla extract make this tea even more delightful!

Little House Tea

Sometimes, when everything becomes too much, we all long to live in a small cottage, a place both cozy and comfortable, where the stress and strain of the outside world seems very far away! I love the simplicity of this tea blend,

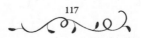

which includes the bright warmth of traditional Earl Grey, and everyone seems to enjoy it.

Simply combine 1 cup Earl Grey tea leaves with 1 tablespoon of crumbled dried lavender blossoms, a few vanilla seeds, and a handful each of dried cornflower and sunflower petals. Store in an airtight jar and use a generous spoonful of the mix to make a cup of comfort tea anytime! If you prefer, you can omit the sunflower petals and use a little dried lemon balm instead.

Safe and Sound Tea

Home is (or should be) a place where we feel safe and protected by positive energies and entities on every level, both physical and emotional. Sadly, sometimes this is not the case and we may need a little extra help; this simple tea blend is always both calming and comforting. Make a cup of this tea for yourself and others when you need to feel surrounded by an aura of true safety without and within. If you use Earl Grey tea instead of the black tea suggested, you will be adding the dimension of protection against illness and health issues of all kinds.

To make a cup of tea, place a teaspoon of light black tea (such as Assam or Darjeeling) in your cup and add 1 teaspoon each dried chamomile tea, dried elderflowers, and a tiny bit of very finely chopped dried lemongrass. Sprin-

kle in a few vanilla seeds. Fill your cup with boiling water, steep for 10 minutes, then strain and drink. Honey adds an extra dimension of protection, too.

Chocolate Chip Shortbread Bars

Shortbread is just one of those cookies that everyone loves; it's also simple to make and keeps well in an airtight container, ready for the next teatime gathering in your warm and inviting kitchen. The chocolate chips are optional but add a little extra flavor burst; they remind me of the wonderful teas I had in Scotland, which is such a magical country steeped in enchantment and tradition. You can use milk or dark chocolate chips, as you prefer.

Preheat oven to 325°F.

Butter a square 8-inch cake pan lightly.

> **1 stick unsalted butter, softened**
> **⅓ cup superfine sugar**
> **1½ cups cake flour**
> **¼ cup cornstarch**
> **¼ teaspoon salt**
> **½ cup chocolate chips**

Cream the butter and sugar together until mixture is light and creamy. In another bowl, sift the flour, cornstarch, and salt together well, then mix this into the butter mixture. Lastly, add the chocolate chips and mix well to

make a soft but not sticky dough. Press the dough evenly into the prepared baking pan and prick lightly with a fork.

Bake for 35–40 minutes, until the shortbread is a pale golden brown. (Don't allow it to become too dark!) Remove from the oven, then cut into squares or bars while still warm. Leave to cool completely in the pan before lifting out the shortbread with an offset spatula. Keeps well for a week at least, but that never seems to actually happen!

MAKES 12–16 BARS OR SQUARES

Little Herb and Cheese Scones

I think smaller is often better when it comes to food served at teatime, and although these scones can be made regular size, I like to use a small 1-inch cutter when making these. You can omit the topping if you prefer and simply serve them with lots of butter and a little extra grated cheese. Use any herbs you like for this recipe—chives, oregano, or parsley also work well.

Preheat oven to 400°F.

Grease a large baking sheet very well.

> 2½ cups flour
> 1 tablespoon baking powder
> ½ teaspoon salt
> ½ cup chilled butter
> A few thyme leaves, chopped

2 tablespoons grated Parmesan
1 egg
2 tablespoons lemon juice
Milk

Sift the flour, baking powder, and salt into a large bowl. Cut the cold butter into small cubes and rub it into the flour until the mixture looks like coarse breadcrumbs. Stir in the chopped herbs and Parmesan. Break the egg into a measuring jug, then add the lemon juice and enough milk to make 1 cup of liquid. Beat briefly, then stir into the flour mixture to make a soft but manageable dough.

Pat the dough out on a floured surface until it is about ½ inch thick and cut out using suitable cutters. (You should be able to get at least 12 2-inch scones or 24 tiny ones out of this recipe.) Place on the baking sheet and bake for 15–20 minutes, until the scones are well risen and golden brown. Cool on a wire rack. Serve warm or cold, but preferably on the day they are made.

Creamy Cheese Topping

Place an 8-ounce package of full fat cream cheese in a bowl and beat until light and fluffy. Stir in a pinch of salt and pepper and ¼ cup sour cream. Lastly, add 2 tablespoons chopped chives or other herb of your choice. Keep the topping refrigerated, and pipe or spoon it on top of the scones just before serving.

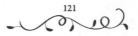

Coronation Chicken Tartlets

Coronation Chicken, a dish of cold chicken served in a lightly curried mayonnaise sauce, comes by its name honestly: it was first served at the coronation of Queen Elizabeth II of Great Britain in 1952. These days it's often served as a filling for teatime sandwiches, but I decided to change things a little and make some little tartlets instead, although this still uses bread as the base, which is easier and quicker than making pastry.

Preheat oven to 350°F.

Grease 10–12 shallow patty pans lightly.

> **10–12 slices soft white bread**
>
> **2 tablespoons butter, melted**
>
> **4 tablespoons olive oil, divided**
>
> **1 small onion, grated**
>
> **1 clove garlic, crushed**
>
> **2 tablespoons chopped red pepper**
>
> **1½ tablespoons mild curry powder**
>
> **1 tablespoon tomato puree**
>
> **2 tablespoons lemon juice**
>
> **¾ cup mayonnaise**
>
> **1½ cups shredded cooked chicken**
>
> **Fresh mint or cilantro**

Use a rolling pin to flatten each slice of bread to about ⅛ inch thick, then use a suitable cutter to cut out circles that will fit in the pans. Combine the melted butter with 2 tablespoons of the oil and brush this mixture lightly on both sides of the bread circles. Press the circles into the patty pans and bake for 15–20 minutes, until the shells are crisp and golden. Cool on a wire rack.

While they are baking, prepare the chicken filling. Heat the remaining olive oil in a saucepan and fry the onion, garlic, and pepper until they are softened and golden. Stir in the curry powder, tomato puree, and lemon juice, and cook to form a paste. Remove from the heat and cool before stirring in the mayonnaise and shredded chicken. Keep refrigerated. Fill the bread shells just before serving, topping each one with a little finely chopped fresh mint or cilantro.

FILLS 10–12 3-INCH TARTLETS

The very least you can do with your life is figure out what you hope for. And the most you can do is live inside that hope.

Barbara Kingsolver

16

Tea in Pyjamas

*I*n general, most of us have a tendency and innate kindness of spirit that makes us put the needs of others before our own; this is, of course, not wrong since caring for those around us—be they immediate family, friends, or the greater community at large—is an essential part of being human. But unfortunately it's safe to say that many of us (and here I have to say that women in particular fall into this category) place our own needs and well-being way down on our to-do list, so far down that they sometimes get totally ignored and forgotten.

Then, after a while, we start to wonder why we are feeling angry, irritable, exhausted, and generally burnt out, which ultimately can lead to an absolute depletion of body, mind, and spirit. In fact, it's my belief, both through personal experience and that of many friends, that physical or

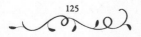

emotional illness often arrive as a wake-up call, a sign that we need to stop doing, worrying, chasing, and enabling and instead let go and give ourselves a chance to simply be. There's a reason why self-care has become a big thing now—because it's needed at this time more than ever before.

Obviously some illnesses do have other causes, and if you have health concerns, they need to be checked out by the relevant health professionals. But sometimes the most pressing need we have is simply to rest, to let go, to retreat; such a beautiful concept. If you ever have the opportunity to go on a retreat, I urge you to do it; they can truly be a life-changing experience. But, since most of us probably can't afford the luxury (and time) for a full-on retreat, I like to think of the concept of tea in pyjamas as a viable and joyful alternative!

Basically, this involves carving out a portion of time (a weekend, a day, a few hours) when you can be quietly with yourself, undisturbed and reflective. And no, it doesn't have to be in pyjamas, just whatever you find comfortable and relaxing to wear. Choose a simple and relaxing place for your quiet time: make sure it's warm if the weather is cold, or perhaps you can choose a quiet outdoor spot on a beautiful summer day. Plan what tea you are going to have—perhaps using some of the recipes in this book—as well as simple, light, nourishing snacks. Gather together all the supplies you need, including cups, teapot, and utensils. Other things that make it special are a few beautiful flowers in a jug or glass, a favorite book to read, your journal, and a fragrant candle. Please do not keep your phone, tablet, or laptop where you can see them all the time; while you may need to stay in contact with others, particularly if you have young children or other family responsibilities, do keep your phone within earshot, just not where you will constantly feel the need to check calls or messages.

Start your quiet time by taking three very deep breaths and allowing yourself to feel the solid earth beneath your feet, the power that holds and nurtures us. Add a little salt and a few drops of lavender or sage essential oil to a cup of water, and use this to purify the space you are in, sprinkling it in all the corners, as well as lightly over your body. Make your tea, then find a comfortable spot to sit or lie down and sip the tea slowly and mindfully, thinking about how you feel. Are you feeling anxious, happy, sad, relaxed? How does your body feel? Light, tired, aching?

If you have a journal, write down any thoughts and emotions that come up for you—without censoring! Who are you on the inside, not the person people think they see

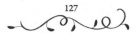

every day? Again, be honest. What do you need to do to be more authentic, to live closer to your truth? Keep sipping your tea and breathing softly and quietly, even if these thoughts and questions make you feel a little anxious.

Then, when the tea is finished, light your candle, gaze at the steady flame for a few moments, and say these words silently or out loud, whichever you prefer.

> *I am here in this precious moment. I am enough just as and who I am. I choose to love and nurture myself now, just as I care for those around me. I choose to give myself time for stillness, for reflection, for healing. I choose to bring myself into the light of my own being, to acknowledge what it is I truly need and desire. I drink this tea with quiet reverence and allow its warmth to flow through me, bringing fresh hope, insight, and joy. And so it is!*

Please note this is also a lovely tea ritual to share with a group of likeminded souls as a wonderful opportunity to get together in a relaxed atmosphere and do a little soul and body nurturing! Choose a couple of hours to spend together—or, even better, a whole day.

Bedtime Teas

The whole concept of "tea in pyjamas" naturally leads us to bedtime, a time of day that should be relaxing in both body and mind but sadly is not always, as some of us battle to fall asleep or let go of the issues or worries of the day! However, it's vitally important that we get good rest after 10 pm, as that is the time of ultimate restorative energy, when the body digests, detoxifies, and rejuvenates.

If, like me, you struggle with falling or staying asleep, here are some simple suggestions for a gentle bedtime ritual that may help. Firstly, remove your phones or other electronic devices and ensure your bedroom is a comfortable temperature, with soft lighting. I like to use candles, but they must be carefully monitored at night to avoid the chance of fire.

Add a few drops of essential oil to an oil burner or diffuser, or simply add them to a little distilled water and sprinkle this mixture on your pillow. Oils particularly suitable for this are lavender, bergamot, geranium, rose, or ylang-ylang. There are a number of tea recipes in this book specifically related to relaxation and better sleep; prepare and slowly sip one. Then lie down flat on your bed, arms relaxed and to the side, hands with palms up. Close your eyes and say the following words very softly:

*Thank you, spirits, for this day, for lessons
learned and gifts given. Tonight I rest
in peace and calm. I am grateful for my
life and all the blessings I have, seen and
unseen. I know my dreams will be joyful,
my sleep calm and restful. And so it is!*

Herb and Turmeric Bedtime Tea

It's often said that a milky drink just before bedtime can help us fall asleep, and this soothing drink is bound to do just that. You can also make it without the milk if you prefer, but it really works better with a dash of creamy milk or nut milk.

Place a teaspoon each of dried lavender blossoms, spearmint, and lemon balm in a large mug, and pour a cup of boiling water over the herbs. Allow to steep for 5–10 minutes, then strain and return the liquid to the mug. Stir in ½ cup warm milk of your choice and a little honey to sweeten. Lastly, stir in ½ teaspoon ground turmeric, which will give the tea a lovely golden color! Serve warm.

Green Healing Tea

This herbal tea holds many gifts in its fragrant warmth—healing, yes, on many levels both physical and emotional, but also protection against negative energies of all kinds as

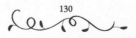

well as creating new and greater abundance in our lives. It's also a powerful antioxidant and very soothing and relaxing to the system.

Put 2 teaspoons of green tea in a cup, then add 1 teaspoon dried chamomile leaves or flowers, 1 teaspoon dried calendula petals, and a few fresh or dried chopped nettle leaves. Pour 1 cup just-boiled water over the herbs, steep for 10–15 minutes, then strain and serve.

Calming Tea

This blend is wonderful for those times when we feel very fearful and stressed. I use it all the time, particularly when I am struggling to get a good night's sleep because of intrusive and anxious thoughts.

Combine 1 cup lemon balm leaves and ½ cup each lavender leaves/flowers, scented geranium leaves, chamomile flowers, and comfrey leaves in a large glass jug (either dried or fresh is fine; use about half as much dried plant material as fresh). Pour 6 cups boiling water over the herbs and steep for 10–15 minutes. Strain and cool before pouring into a jug. Drink one cup of the warmed liquid as needed; store the rest in the fridge, where it will keep for 3–4 days.

An excellent alternative herbal tea for peaceful and calm sleep is made with 2 parts chamomile flowers and 1 part each dried lavender blossoms/leaves and dried valerian root.

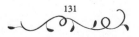

Clearing and Refreshing Tea

No matter what the time of year, we can all suffer from the misery of colds, flu, hay fever, and other issues that leave us miserable and depleted. This is a simple herbal tea blend that can be stored and taken at the onset of any of these conditions.

Place 1 teaspoon each dried thyme and sage leaves (crumbled) in the bottom of your teacup, then add a tiny piece of fresh chopped ginger root and 1 teaspoon finely grated fresh lemon zest. Pour 1 cup just-boiled water over the herbs and steep for 10 minutes. Strain and serve with a drop of honey and a thin slice of lemon.

Immunitea Blend

We often need to increase our levels of immunity, especially at times of stress or physical exhaustion for whatever reason; a healthy immune system is our strongest defence against the onset of illness, either chronic or acute. The ingredients in this blend all have proven health and immunity benefits and are associated with healing and protection on all levels: physical, emotional, and spiritual.

For a cup of joyful health and immunity, combine the following: 1 teaspoon green tea (or matcha), 1 teaspoon each dried calendula petals and dried elderflowers, ½ teaspoon ground turmeric, and a little finely grated fresh or dried orange rind. Pour 1 cup just-boiled water over the herbs, stir very well, and steep for 5 minutes, then strain and serve. As you sip this aromatic blend, feel its warmth and light filling and healing you from the inside out.

Sunshine Lemon Bars

Sweet and sassy at the same time, these bar cookies offer us the bright warmth of lemon and the courage of thyme, reminding us to nurture and honor the gift that is our unique body and spirit. If you have lemon thyme, that would be perfect here!

Preheat oven to 350°F.

Grease a 9-inch square baking pan well.

> 1 stick unsalted butter, softened
> ½ cup sugar
> 1½ cups cake flour, sifted
> ½ cup finely shredded coconut
> ½ teaspoon salt
> 1 14-ounce can sweetened condensed milk
> 1 egg
> ⅔ cup fresh lemon juice
> Finely grated zest of 1 lemon
> 1 tablespoon chopped thyme leaves

Cream the butter and sugar together until fluffy and light, then stir in the flour, coconut, and salt, mixing well

to form a fairly firm dough. Take about one-third of the dough, form it into a ball, and place in the refrigerator. Press the remaining two-thirds of the dough evenly over the base of the prepared baking pan, prick lightly with a fork, and bake for 5–10 minutes or until just golden. Leave to cool in the pan.

To make the filling, whisk together the condensed milk, egg, lemon juice, and zest; the mixture will thicken a bit. Spread this evenly over the cooled pastry base and sprinkle the finely chopped thyme leaves over the top, then grate the chilled portion of the dough over the filling. Bake for 25–30 minutes or until the topping is just golden brown. Leave to cool in the pan, then dust with confectioners' sugar and cut into bars or squares to serve. These keep well for a few days in an airtight container.

MAKES ABOUT 16 BARS

Almond-Orange Biscotti

I grew up in South Africa, where everyone eats rusks. For breakfast, with tea, as a quick snack—you name it. However, my Italian father (who never drank tea but only coffee, as dark and strong as possible) refused to refer to them as rusks and instead called them by their Italian name of biscotti. They are both simple and delicious, whatever you choose to call them, and seem particularly suited to a relaxing tea at home. Another advantage is that you can swap out flavors to suit yourself: lemon instead of orange, pecans or walnuts, dried fruit, chocolate chips, snipped herbs like lemon balm or lavender...

Preheat oven to 350°F.

Line a large cookie sheet with baking paper.

> **2 cups flour**
> **1½ teaspoons baking powder**
> **¼ teaspoon salt**
> **½ cup flaked almonds**
> **1 stick unsalted butter, softened**
> **¾ cup sugar**
> **2 eggs, beaten**
> **¼ cup fresh orange juice**
> **Grated zest of one orange**

Sift the flour, baking powder, and salt together, and then stir in the flaked almonds. In a large bowl, cream the butter and sugar together until light and fluffy, then add the eggs, orange juice, and zest. Mix well before stirring in the dry ingredients and beat to form a soft dough. Turn the dough out on the cookie sheet and shape into a log measuring approximately 3 inches wide by 15 inches long. Bake in the preheated oven for 20–25 minutes, by which time the log should be light golden brown and firm to the touch. Remove from the oven and cool on the baking sheet.

Use a serrated knife to carefully cut the cooled log into around 16 to 18 slices; cut slightly on the diagonal for the best results. Place the slices back onto the cookie sheet and bake again for another 10 minutes. (This gives the biscotti their traditional crisp texture.) Cool completely before storing in an airtight container; these cookies keep very well and as such are perfect for easy tea entertaining or spur-of-the-moment get-togethers.

Honey-Banana Scones

Honey and banana flavor these soft, light scones with warmth and sweetness and also infuse them with all their healing properties, such as healing and prosperity (honey) and spirituality and fertility (banana). These are best served warm, preferably with butter and a little more golden honey.

Preheat oven to 400°F.

Grease a large baking sheet well.

  3 cups flour
  4 teaspoons baking powder
  ½ teaspoon salt
  2 tablespoons sugar
  ½ teaspoon ground nutmeg
  ½ stick chilled unsalted butter
  1 large ripe banana

2 tablespoons honey

1 egg

½ cup buttermilk

Sift the flour, baking powder, salt, sugar, and nutmeg together in a large bowl, then cut the butter into small pieces and rub in with your fingers until the mixture resembles large breadcrumbs. In another bowl, mash the peeled banana very well, then stir in the honey, egg, and buttermilk. Add this to the flour mixture and beat well until a soft but manageable dough is formed.

Press the dough out gently on a floured surface—it should be about ¾–1 inch thick. Using a cookie or scone cutter, cut out rounds and place the scones on the prepared baking sheet. Bake for 10–12 minutes or until the scones are well risen and light golden-brown. Cool on a wire rack and serve as fresh as possible!

MAKES 10–12 SCONES

When I walk, I walk
with you. Where I go,
you're with me always.

Alice Hoffman

17

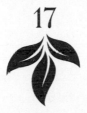

A Faerie Goddess Tea

rowing up, we were fortunate enough to have a truly beautiful and magical garden full of trees, flowers, and green beauty, as well as lots of little paths and interesting nooks and crannies. I believed then, and still do, that faeries came to play in that lovely garden among the birds, butterflies, and ladybugs! My mother gave lots of memorable tea parties when I was a little girl, but particularly magical were the faerie tea parties she occasionally created as a special birthday treat for me and my friends. I had one of those tiny china tea sets sprinkled with roses, and I remember she made little cups of jasmine and rose tea in them, as well as miniature cakes with pink frosting.

But faeries are not just for children and storybooks and Disney movies, they are for all of us, whoever and wherever we are, as a bright, beautiful reminder of the potential for

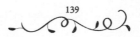

joy and enchantment we can all find in our everyday lives. No matter how old we are, we can open ourselves to the light, wisdom, and blessings of the faeries, and what better way than by creating a magical tea in their honor?

Simple moments of finding joy in just being alive are the ultimate gifts of the faerie beings to us. And teatime is a liminal time, a time between worlds and everyday realities, so it's the perfect introduction and opening to faerie worlds, too. They remind us that we carry shining magic within ourselves, and it's this enchantment we can bring into our lives and ways of being every day. (Please remember that if you notice ladybugs in your garden, it's a clear sign of the fae being present, as they adore ladybugs and are often said to keep them as pets!)

Faeries love cakes, milk, honey, and all small, sweet offerings, so these should be a part of your faerie tea. And they also obviously adore lots of color, sparkles, and flowers, so make your tables as bright and pretty as you can!

This is a simple blessing and welcome you can share to encourage the faeries' presence at your tea table:

> *In this beautiful moment, all blessings*
> *and magic are ours. We have chosen to*
> *step away from the everyday world to*
> *another place—an enchanted place, a place*
> *where we can play with the faeries and*

remember the magic within. This magic
is always with us, and we ask the faeries
to join us in this simple celebration of
happiness and inspiration. And so it is!

Faerie Sprinkles

This fragrant sprinkle mixture, which is rather akin to a simple potpourri, can be placed in small bowls on the tea table or added to tiny glass bottles that are then tied up with small, bright ribbons and beads to make faerie wish bottles—a lovely party favor or gift.

You will need a handful of dried lavender leaves or blossoms and the same of pine needles, and a little dried rosemary and sage. Mix in a small bowl, then add 6 drops sandalwood essential oil and 2 drops rose essential oil. Add 1 tablespoon pink Himalayan salt crystals and mix well. You can also add some dried flower petals, such as rose, cornflower, or marigold, for a bright burst of color. This mixture will keep for a few weeks and has lots of magical and protective properties, just like the faeries themselves!

Seeing the Faeries Tea and Magic Wash

If you want to see the faeries, you will do well to employ this delicate tea mix, which can also be used to make a magic wash to lightly sprinkle around yourself and your garden or home.

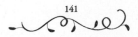

It's very simple to make. You take some hibiscus flowers, a handful of marigold petals, and the same of thyme leaves, and pour a cup of just-boiled water over them. Add a handful of dried rose petals and a few drops of rose flower essence if you have it. Drink as a tea or allow it to cool and use the liquid as a beautiful and enchanted wash for body and home.

Faerie Wishes Tea Blend

Will this fragrant tea blend help your wishes come true? Only the faeries know the answer to that one, but sipping this tea certainly won't hurt—and remember to pour a little into a tiny cup and leave it for the winged ones to enjoy too! This fragrant tea blend also encourages positivity and a sunny outlook.

For a dried tea blend, mix together the following and store in an airtight glass jar: 2 parts dried chamomile leaves or flowers, 1 part each green tea leaves, lemon balm, and calendula petals, and a handful of dried rose petals. Use 2 teaspoons of this blend per cup of hot water, steep for 10 minutes, then strain and serve. A little dried lemon zest can be sprinkled on top of the tea, too. Sip slowly and be open to the whispers and encouragement of the faerie folk around you, even if they are choosing to remain invisible!

Borage Tea Cooler

Faeries, as well as bees and butterflies, love the bright and beautiful flowers of borage, and we can all benefit from the positive message of joy and courage linked to this ancient herb. This is an iced tea blend that is wonderful for serving at summertime teas in the garden.

Place 2 cups of borage leaves in a large jug and add the rind and juice of 1 large lemon. Add 6 cloves and a handful of fresh mint leaves. Pour 5–6 cups just boiled water over the herbs, steep for 10 minutes, then strain and allow to get cold. Dilute with either sparkling mineral water or unsweetened apple juice before serving with lots of ice and garnished with fresh borage flowers.

Dandelion Divination Tea

In order to see the faeries and their enchanted realms, we need to look with the inner eyes of our heart and soul and see beyond seeing, as it is sometimes said. The two flower ingredients of this simple, fresh tea are both linked to the powers of divination and the opening up of new and different portals of possibility.

Simply place a handful each of fresh dandelion petals and leaves and marigold petals in your cup and pour a cup of just-boiled water over them. Add a slice of fresh orange

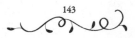

or lemon and allow the mixture to steep for 5 minutes. Strain and serve sweetened with honey.

Magic Realms Meditation Tea

Another simple tea blend to use at faerie tea celebrations or indeed anytime you would like to be in a quietly receptive mood for magic and meditation. These three ingredients are linked with inspiration, positive energies, and the flow of beauty and joy through and in our beings.

For a cup you will need 2 teaspoons dried mint or spearmint, 1 teaspoon dried chamomile flowers (or open a chamomile tea bag and use that), and a sprinkling of dried, fragrant rose petals. Pour 1 cup of just-boiled water over the herbs, steep for 5 minutes, strain, and serve while inhaling the peaceful fragrance of your tea and allowing it to permeate your being on every level.

Strawberry Meringue Bars

Faeries are particularly fond of berries of all kinds, so these little bar cookies are the perfect addition to your faerie goddess tea menu. You can use other preserves if you prefer, such as blackberry or raspberry.

Preheat oven to 350°F.

Grease an 8-inch square baking pan very well.

1½ cups shredded sweetened coconut

2 egg whites

1 cup butter, softened

¾ cup sugar

2 cups cake flour

1 cup strawberry preserves

Mix the coconut and egg whites in a small bowl and set aside. Cream the butter and sugar until the mixture is light and fluffy, then slowly beat in the flour to make a firm but manageable dough. Press the dough evenly over the base of the baking pan and prick all over with a fork. Bake for 25 minutes or until a pale golden color.

Remove from the oven and spread the jam on top, followed by the coconut mixture. Return to the oven and bake for a further 15 minutes. Cool in the pan and cut into squares or bars. They keep well in an airtight container for a few days.

MAKES 12–16 SQUARES OR BARS

Creamy Mint and Cucumber Sandwiches

Green and fresh, these are an update on the cucumber sandwiches traditionally served at afternoon teas. I remember my mother making them and even non-cucumber-lovers really enjoyed them, but perhaps it was her delicious homemade mayonnaise! I consider them to be the perfect food for a faerie tea since the fae love green in all its shades

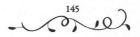

and permutations. You will see that this recipe is fairly flexible and non-prescriptive; the only essential is soft white bread, as these sandwiches lose some of their delicacy when made with brown or whole wheat bread.

> **1 or 2 medium cucumbers**
> **12 slices fresh white bread**
> **Unsalted butter, softened**
> **1 cup mayonnaise**
> **2 teaspoons lemon juice**
> **A handful of fresh mint**
> **A few fresh chives**
> **Ground paprika (optional)**

First, peel the cucumbers and slice them very thinly. Place on paper towels for a little while—this absorbs moisture and stops the sandwiches from becoming soggy.

Remove the crusts from the bread and spread six slices thinly with softened butter. Combine the mayonnaise with the lemon juice and spread a thin layer on top of the butter. Arrange the cucumber slices on top of this, then scatter the mint and chives over the top. Dust with ground paprika if you like. Cover with the remaining slices of bread, carefully cut each sandwich into four quarters, then arrange on a serving plate and cover with plastic wrap. Refrigerate until just before serving; they should be as cool as the proverbial cucumber!

MAKES 24 SMALL SANDWICH QUARTERS

Butterfly Cakes

A traditional and beautiful way of turning everyday cupcakes into something a little magical! You can substitute a teaspoon of rose water for the vanilla or sprinkle a tablespoon of very finely chopped lavender blossoms into the batter.

Preheat oven to 350°F.

Grease 12 muffins pans well or line with paper liners.

> **1 stick unsalted butter, softened**
>
> **1 cup sugar**
>
> **2 eggs**
>
> **1 teaspoon vanilla extract**
>
> **1½ cups cake flour**
>
> **2 teaspoons baking powder**
>
> **½ teaspoon salt**
>
> **½ cup buttermilk**

Cream the butter and sugar together until light and fluffy. Beat the eggs and add to the butter mixture, together with the vanilla extract. Sift together the flour, baking powder, and salt, and stir into the butter mixture, alternately with the buttermilk, until you have a smooth and creamy batter. Divide this between the prepared muffin pans and bake for 20–25 minutes or until the cupcakes are well risen and light golden-brown. Cool on a wire rack.

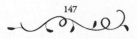

When the cakes are cold, use a sharp knife to slice off the domed top of each cupcake, and cut this in half. Spread or pipe frosting on the top of the cupcake, then arrange the two pieces of cake at an angle from each other to resemble wings. Decorate as you like: pastel-colored sprinkles or dusting sugar or use a few fresh blossoms, such as lavender or tiny thyme flowers.

Faerie Frosting

Beat together 1 stick softened unsalted butter with 2 cups confectioners' sugar until light and fluffy. Add a little flavoring of your choice, such as vanilla extract or rose water. You may need to add a little extra sugar if the frosting becomes too runny. Pink frosting would look lovely; add a tablespoon of fresh raspberry or strawberry puree to the frosting or check out other natural frosting options online.

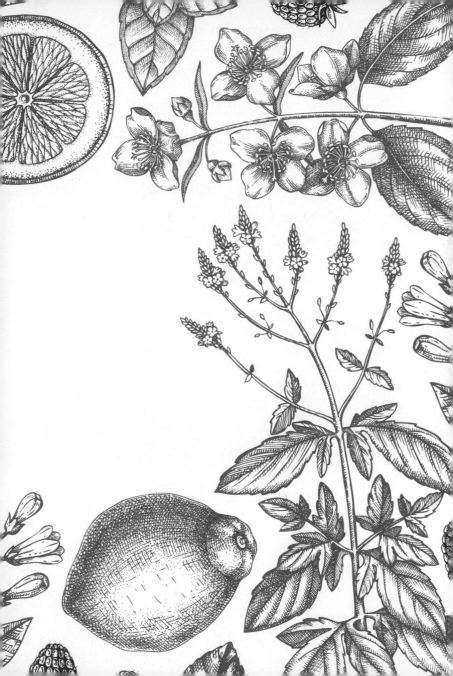

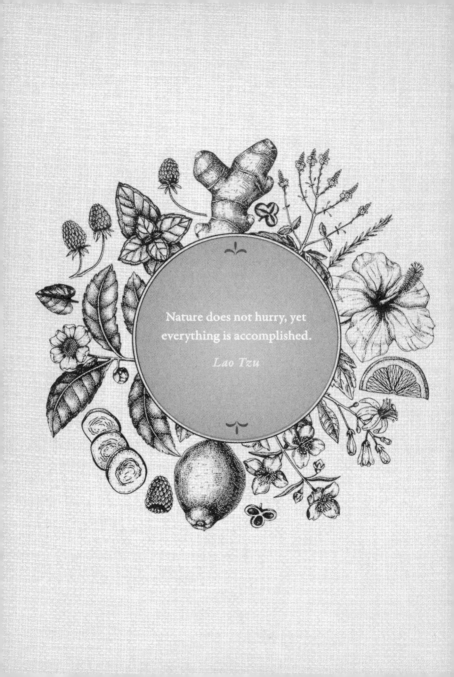

Nature does not hurry, yet
everything is accomplished.

Lao Tzu

18

A Wild Green Tea

Whoever we are, wherever we live, whatever we do, our inborn nature is wild … as much so as the winds and waters, the birds and butterflies, and the trees and flowers. We are at once from and of the earth, our beautiful and nurturing womb and home. Yet we can forget this truth, either knowingly or unconsciously, as we attempt to navigate our way through what can sometimes seem increasingly noisy and complicated lives.

Perhaps we need to tap into the innate life force that surrounds us again—the life force that offers us all peace, hope, and healing of body and spirit. Paradise is not far away in some mystical realm or future; it's right here, all around us. We just need to learn (again?) to see it, honor it, and, above all, become part of it.

You may well be asking what this has to do with tea. The teas we drink, whether for health, magic, or simple enjoyment, are filled with earth's gifts too and become a part of our being in much the same way as the earth is. For it is in the wild spaces and also in cultivated gardens that we are closest to our wild, unfettered selves—selves that we often (women in particular) put aside along the way in our attempt to fill roles and preordained patterns—sometimes imposed on us by the expectations of others, sometimes by our own desire to fit in and not rock any boats!

These days few of us can be unfamiliar with the Japanese concept of *shinrin-yoku*, or forest bathing. This is both a calming and healing ritual that simply involves spending time quietly in a forest or other green space, walking slowly or sitting in quiet thought while we allow our surroundings to work their magic on our bodies and minds. It's been proven that plants give off chemicals called phytoncides, which help to heal and balance our immune system. We feel more connected and less stressed, our breathing slows, and our blood pressure goes down.

There's a beautiful Japanese phrase that may be translated as "flower bird wind moon"; basically it means the contemplation of the beauty of nature and thereby our own beauty and magnificence. We can find our true rhythm in wild green spaces and remember who and what we truly are.

Here are some thoughts and ideas from a wild green tea/ceremony I created last year in early summer:

Firstly, I admit I am very lucky in that I live in a wild green space—and I only have to step outside to already find myself in the middle of a forest! It seemed to be the perfect place to invite a small group of like-minded friends to spend the morning in thought, meditation, and the sharing of tea—a simple celebration of the earth, her beauty, and ourselves. We started the wild green tea with an hour spent walking the grounds or sitting and lying on the earth in silence; no phones allowed! Barefoot and in loose, comfortable clothing, we allowed ourselves to absorb the sounds, smells, and energies of the earth all around us. I also suggested people could bring a small notebook and pen to record any thoughts or emotions that might arise during this time.

Later we gathered at a long wooden table on which I had arranged cups and a few small bowls containing different dried herbs. There was a small label on each bowl indicating the name of the herb and its healing or magical properties. I suggested that each member of the group think about what herbal tea would be most meaningful or helpful to them at this current time in their life and then mix an appropriate blend in their cup.

I then added some freshly boiled spring water to their cups. I would like to say I made a fire to boil the water by rubbing two sticks together, but the truth is I actually brought a small gas burner from my home for this task; I like to simplify things when I can! We sat and sipped our teas in quiet thought and contemplation, and then we shared a few thoughts about what this time had meant and how we felt we could be more fully wild in our lives.

We also ate a few simple earth-based snacks—further evidence of the many gifts we receive from our green mother every day.

To end the morning, we stood around the table holding hands and said the following words together:

> *As we stand and walk and move in this*
> *beautiful place, we remember how we are*
> *blessed every day by the spirit of our Mother*
> *Earth and her gentle wisdom and guidance.*
> *We are reminded of our wildness and that we*
> *are free and full of possibility. Like the flowers*
> *and trees, we are growing and blooming in*
> *our magnificence. Like the birds, we have a*
> *song to sing. Like the butterflies, we can soar.*
> *Above all, we can honor ourselves and our*
> *wild spirits every day we have on this magical*
> *and green earth. Blessed be. And so it is!*

Of course you can use this tea ritual when you are alone, too—in fact, I find that sometimes the greatest impact of forest bathing comes when we walk in solitude and silence, open to the inner words of the heart.

Rose Verbena Tea

Such a simple and delicate tea for quiet moments in nature—even the soft colors of green and rose are a beautiful reminder of the garden's gifts. Apparently it's helpful for indigestion, but to be perfectly honest this is just a tea I love in its gentle simplicity; I always keep a jar of the blend in my pantry and take a flask of the tea with me on days spent in gardens and forests.

You will need 1 cup Chinese green tea, ½ cup dried rose petals or buds, and ¼ cup dried lemon verbena leaves. Simply mix these together with your hands, then store the tea in an airtight jar or tin. Use 1 heaped tablespoon for a pot of tea (3–4 cups).

Green Ritual Tea

This recipe was originally developed for use with full moon rituals, but these days I find its herb and flower magic ideal for any time spent out of doors in green places. It is just beautiful and uplifting on every level, for heart and mind. Drink it slowly and mindfully when you are in a garden

or forest and open yourself to the messages you are receiving all around from the plants, trees, birds, and other little creatures sharing this space.

To make a cup of this magical tea, combine a handful of fresh elderflowers with 2–3 lavender sprigs, 1 jasmine tea bag, ½ teaspoon dried yarrow leaves, and 3 crushed cardamom pods. Pour 1 cup just-boiled water over the herbs, steep for 5–10 minutes, then strain and serve sweetened with honey.

Green Spirit Tea

Often by the time we realize we need to get back to our roots (so to speak) and find our own wild green hearts again, we are already burnt out, dispirited, and lacking joy in our lives. This tea—which again uses my favorite herbal tea ally, green tea—provides a gentle lift and antidote to this sad and empty mood.

For each cup, you will need one green tea bag to which you add 1 tablespoon dried rose petals and 1 teaspoon each dried dandelion leaves and finely chopped dried nettle. Pour 1 cup of just-boiled water over the herbs, steep for 10 minutes, then strain and serve with a cinnamon stick.

Simple Herb & Fruit Infusions

These simple, refreshing, and cleansing cold infusions are prepared the night before and carried with you on your wild green travels. In every case, combine the sliced fruit and chopped herbs (or other ingredients) in a large glass jug, pour 1½ pints spring or mineral water over the herbs, cover the jug, and leave it in the refrigerator overnight.

Try the following combinations:

- Cucumber, sliced lemon, and finely chopped basil leaves

- Orange, chopped mint, and fennel seeds

- Blackberries and fresh sage leaves

- Apple slices, a few sprigs of rosemary, and a little cinnamon

Caraway Flatbreads with Pesto

A plate of these small breads topped with homemade pesto makes the perfect addition to a wild green tea, and the beauty of making your own pesto is that you can choose your own favorite herbs or use ones that seem particularly appropriate to the occasion. You can make the flatbreads up to five days in advance and store them in an airtight container.

Preheat oven to 325°F.

Grease 1 or 2 large baking sheets well.

2 cups flour, sifted

1 teaspoon baking powder

2 teaspoons caraway seeds

½ teaspoon sea salt flakes

¼ cup plain yoghurt

¼ cup olive oil

Combine the flour, baking powder, caraway seeds, and salt in a large bowl. Add the yoghurt and olive oil and mix with your hands, adding just enough cold water to form a soft but not sticky dough. When the dough is smooth and well combined, roll it out on a floured surface until it's about ¼-inch thick and cut out circles about 2 inches in diameter. Arrange the circles on the baking sheets—you may need to bake the breads in batches—and bake for 5 minutes or until the flatbreads are pale golden and crisp. Top each of the flatbreads with a spoonful of pesto (see next recipe) just before serving. These breads are also great served with dips and soups.

Pesto Magic 101

I love making pesto and adapting it to suit a particular event or just what I have in my garden. Although pesto traditionally includes nuts, I don't usually include them as so many of the people I know are allergic—however, you can always add a small handful of finely chopped pine nuts,

pecans, or almonds, if you choose. You do really need a food processor or blender to make pesto, but if you have lots of energy you can also use a pestle and mortar.

To make one of my favorite pestos, you will need 1 cup each fresh basil leaves and fresh flat-leaved parsley and 3 peeled and chopped fresh garlic cloves. Place these in a food processor and pulse until finely chopped; add the grated zest of a small lemon, approximately ½ cup olive oil, and ¼ cup finely grated Parmesan cheese. Process until the pesto is well amalgamated and fairly smooth—there should be no large leaves or bits of stem in the mixture. Taste and add a little salt and pepper if needed, then place in an airtight jar and store in the refrigerator. It can be kept for a couple of weeks.

Other herbs that work well in pesto are chives, cilantro, or mint. You can also add a chopped green or red chili to the mix if you would like a spicier version. For a wild green version, use chopped nettles in place of the parsley.

Japanese Cheesecake

This delicate crustless cheesecake is light and gently perfumed with green tea and jasmine flavors. In Japan there are many versions of this treat, but this is the one I think is the most suitable tribute to forest bathing, an essential part of any wild green life (and tea)! Please use a full-fat cream

cheese for this, and also note that you can use vanilla or lemon as a flavoring if you prefer. The cheesecake is baked in a water bath to ensure it retains its soft and creamy texture, so you will need a fairly deep ovenproof dish to stand the cake pan in while baking.

Preheat oven to 350°F.

Line a deep 7- or 8-inch cake pan and grease well.

- **½ cup milk or light cream**
- **2 each green tea and jasmine tea bags**
- **8 ounces soft cream cheese**
- **⅔ cup superfine sugar**
- **5 eggs, separated**
- **2 tablespoons butter**
- **2 tablespoons cake flour**
- **1 tablespoon cornstarch**
- **1 tablespoon lemon juice**

Warm the milk or cream gently with the tea bags to allow the flavors to infuse. Strain the liquid and mix with the cream cheese to make a smooth mixture. Beat the sugar and egg yolks together and add to the cream cheese mixture. Stir in the butter, flour, and cornstarch, and beat well. In another bowl beat the 5 egg whites with the lemon juice until stiff but not dry; gently fold into the cream cheese batter. Pour the batter into the prepared cake pan and wrap two layers of aluminum foil around the outside to prevent any water from getting into the pan. Place a deep oven dish of hot water in the oven, and carefully set the cake pan into it. Bake for 30–35 minutes, then lower the oven temperature to 325°F and continue baking for another 20–25 minutes. The cheesecake should look golden, risen, and lightly firm to the touch. Leave to cool in the pan and remove carefully only once fully cold. Refrigerate until serving; this cheesecake is wonderful served with a little whipped cream and some lemon curd or fresh berries on the side.

SERVES 6–8

Green Magic Bars

These are probably one of the most delicious and simple things to make in this book! They are the perfect addition to a tea in the wild, as they are easily transported and keep well. This is also a very flexible recipe as you can mix and match the ingredients to suit personal taste and what you have available in your kitchen. I like to use almonds, macadamias, and shelled pistachios for their pretty pop of green color.

Grease or line an 8-inch-square cake pan with baking paper.

> ½ cup chopped mixed nuts
> ⅛ cup honey or maple syrup
> ¼ cup dried fruit, chopped

161

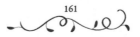

1 cup shredded dried coconut

1 cup rolled oats (not instant)

Pinch of salt

½ teaspoon ground cardamom

¼ cup coconut oil

Basically, all you need to do is place all the ingredients, apart from the coconut oil, in a large bowl and mix well. Gently warm the coconut oil and then pour it over the dry ingredients and mix until a sticky dough is formed—a messy business, but keep going! You may need to add a little warm water to ensure you have a dough that holds together. Press the dough into the prepared cake pan and refrigerate while you make the topping.

Topping

In a small saucepan, warm together ⅓ cup honey or maple syrup, ¼ cup raw cacao powder, ½ teaspoon vanilla extract, and ⅓ cup coconut oil. When the mixture is well combined and thick, remove from the heat. Allow to cool before spreading on the nut bars. Sprinkle with a few finely chopped herbs of your choice (possibly mint, lemon balm, or thyme) or sprinkle with crushed dried lavender blossoms. Cut into bars or squares and keep in an airtight container until serving.

MAKES 12–16 SQUARES OR BARS

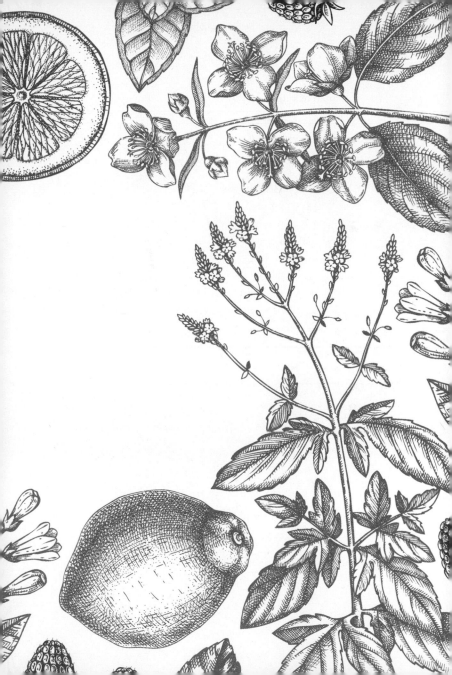

Wherever you go, no matter
what the weather, always
bring your own sunshine.

Anthony J. D'Angelo

19

Tea in the Garden

*J*ust being in a garden is both healing and an adventure for all our senses. An oasis and sanctuary for mind, body, and spirit, in the garden there is color, fragrance, sound, taste, and the warmth of the sun for our blessing and enchantment. For us kitchen witches, the garden is an extension of our home and hearth—a place where we can use and celebrate earth's bounty in the form of flowers, herbs, fruits, leaves, and more.

I personally think taking tea among the flowers is the single most beautiful thing one can do—and even if we don't have a personal garden space, I hope that you will be able to find a public garden that can become a place of rejuvenation and peace for you. A garden is also a sacred and healing space where the mind becomes open and more responsive to nature's gentle magic. Flowers, herbs, trees,

and other plants really do possess so many spiritual, meta-physical, and practical properties that can enrich our lives on every level.

Tea among the flowers can, of course, be as simple as packing a flask of hot tea (or a jug of iced) and a few cookies or sandwiches and carrying these into our garden space, either alone or with a few special people. In fact, picnic teas in the garden are a lovely idea in general, with each person being given their own little box or basket with a mug, tea bag, and a few bite-sized tea treats. A friend of mine uses metal Japanese bento boxes for this, which also work very well and have the advantage of being both sturdy and reusable.

Tea among the flowers can also be a truly magical way of celebrating a special occasion such as a birthday, a new baby, or a wedding. Recently, on a wonderfully sunny and warm late summer afternoon, I attended a handfasting held in a beautiful wild garden not far from my home.

It was so natural and beautiful with wooden tables and chairs, pottery mugs and platters of simple foods, and jugs of wildflowers—daisies, dandelions, wild roses, and herbs of all kinds. Some of these flowers were also scattered around the place where the couple stood to make their commitment to each other. After the ceremony we sat, talked, and listened to some quiet music, and before we knew it the shadows were lengthening on the grass and the afternoon was almost gone ...

As a final gift, the flowers were gathered into small bunches, tied with bright ribbons, and given to the departing guests. I still have mine, dried, in an old blue jug. It's a reminder of how simple moments can become lasting memories.

Even if you don't have a particular occasion to celebrate today, why not celebrate the joy of being alive on this beautiful green earth of ours? Take a few flowers or herbs and scatter them around the place where you will be taking tea. Sit quietly (either singly or as a group) and breathe slowly and with intention for a few moments. Before you take tea, share any thoughts, prayers, or wishes you may have. You can also write in your journal at this time. Eat and drink mindfully, taking notice of your surroundings—birds and their song, butterflies and droning bees, the color and fragrance of the plants.

When the tea is finished, give thanks:

The garden heals us on so many levels.
We are truly grateful for this brief moment
of time and beauty. We are here. All is as
it should be. We are blessed. And so it is!

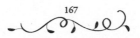

Finally, take a few small reminders of the day—perhaps a fallen leaf or a smooth pebble. And don't forget to pour a few drops of tea at the base of a nearby tree, giving thanks for the gifts of the garden. If there is a source of running water, like a stream, in the garden, sprinkle a few leaves or blossoms in it and allow the flowing water to carry your wishes and dreams to the source and mother of us all.

Making Tussie-Mussies

These little posies make the perfect table decoration for a floral tea and can be given to each guest to take home as a reminder of a beautiful day. Originally tussie-mussies were carried in medieval times to not only ward off the noxious smells that were a part of everyday life, but also to confer protection against illness and disease. Endless variations of herbs and flowers can be used to make these bouquets, but they should all be as fragrant as possible.

The centre is usually a highly scented rose (or possibly a few fragrant violets) around which are placed feathery silver leaves such as artemisia or lavender; the bouquet is then tied firmly with cotton twine. Continue to build up the circles of the tussie mussie with a circle of mint or lavender and then a circle of lemon balm, sage, or rosemary. Finish off with a circle of scented geranium leaves and then tie the whole bouquet tightly. Stand the tussie mussies in

little glasses of water to keep them fresh. They also dry well and can be kept for a long time, especially if a little suitable essential oil is added to revitalize the fragrance.

Garden Tea of Provence

Make up a batch of this delicate floral tea that is based on the traditional herbes de Provence mixture and serve it in a garden. The flowers and herbs will bring about a gentle sense of well-being, peace, and beauty!

This recipe is given in parts so you can adapt it to suit your personal needs; it keeps well in a jar or tin. Combine two parts dried oregano or marjoram and two parts dried and crumbled lavender leaves and flowers with one part each dried rosemary, thyme, and rose petals. Add a sprinkling of dried fennel seeds and use to make tea in the proportions of 1½ teaspoons to 1 cup boiling water.

Rooibos, Honey, and Mint Iced Tea

With or without an extra kick, this is a refreshing tea drink for summer occasions or serving outdoors. I find rooibos tea quite strong and dominant on its own, so I prefer it mixed with other herbs and ingredients.

In a jug, steep 4 rooibos tea bags in 3 cups boiling water for at least 10 minutes. Strain and add honey to taste. When the tea is cold, pour it into a large glass jug and add

4 cups sparkling water. Chill well. Just before serving, stir in ½ cup Southern Comfort (optional) and a handful of crushed mint leaves. Stir and serve with ice.

MAKES ABOUT 7 CUPS ICED TEA

Gardener's Healing Tea

Gardening is lovely, but no one can deny it takes a heavy toll on muscles and joints! This recipe, which is wonderfully soothing for painful backs and hands, has been adapted from Cerridwen Greenleaf's lovely *Book of Kitchen Witchery*. Again, I have given the recipe in parts so you can adjust it to suit the quantities of dried herb you have.

Mix two parts each dried echinacea and chamomile with one part dried mint and one part each dried anise seeds and dried thyme leaves. Store this mixture in an airtight jar or tin and add 1–2 teaspoons to a cup of boiling water. Steep for 10 minutes, strain, and serve, sweetened with a little stevia or honey if you like. This makes both a soothing and energising tisane after a long day in the garden.

Potpourri Tea

Potpourri, or the use of dried or fresh herbs, flowers, and other fragrant plants to make scented mixtures for the home, is an ancient art and one that has gotten something of a negative rap in the past few decades, owing to the

proliferation of some truly horrible and false commercial products masquerading under the name. However, the making of true potpourri is a lovely green tradition and one we should all try at least once in our lives—but in the meantime, here is a recipe for a simple tea that brings us garden healing and positive energies from the spices and the beauty of hibiscus.

This herbal tea blend may be stored in airtight tins or jars for up to six months. You will need ½ cup light black tea leaves, 1 broken cinnamon stick, 2 star anise, 5 cloves, 1 tablespoon dried hibiscus flowers, and the dried peel of a small orange. Combine these ingredients well and store as suggested above. Use 1–2 teaspoons of the blend to make a cup of tea with 1 cup of just-boiled water.

Sweet Romance Tea

Sometimes we all feel a little unloved, or as if we need some extra passion in our lives—but please note, this is *not* a tea designed to attract someone! We all know that love spells are not generally a good idea because the only love worth having is that which is both freely offered and received. Rather, this tea helps us to see our own innate worthiness of love and affection despite whatever may be happening in our outward circumstances, and ultimately that will make us attract the souls most in tune with our personal being.

(Please note that this tea should be avoided if you are pregnant because raspberry leaf is a uterine stimulant.)

To make one cup, place 1 teaspoon of white tea in your cup (or use a tea bag); add 1 teaspoon each dried raspberry leaf and lemon balm leaves and a few scented rose petals. (You can also add a few drops of vanilla extract if you like, but be sparing with it as it can easily dominate all other flavors.) Pour 1 cup of just-boiled water over the herbs, steep for 5 minutes, then strain and serve.

Almond-Raspberry Swirls

When I lived in London, I used to go to a small bakery on cold, wet mornings and order something very similar to these, although my version is made without yeast. These light pastries with their sweet raspberry filling make the ideal accompaniment for your garden tea!

Preheat oven to 400°F.

Line a large baking sheet with baking paper and grease lightly.

> **2 cups cake flour**
> **4 teaspoons baking powder**
> **½ teaspoon salt**
> **½ stick butter, chilled**
> **1 egg**
> **1 cup buttermilk**

1 cup raspberry preserves
¼ cup flaked almonds for garnish

Glaze

Mix ½ cup confectioners' sugar with 1 teaspoon almond or vanilla extract and enough warm water to make a thick yet spreadable mixture.

Combine flour, baking powder, and salt in a large bowl and either grate or chop the butter into the flour mixture. Beat egg and buttermilk together and then stir into the flour mixture to make a soft dough. Press the dough out on a floured board to make a rectangle about 8 × 10 inches that is ½-inch thick.

For the filling, spread the raspberry preserves evenly over the dough, then roll up carefully from the long side and press together firmly. Use a sharp knife to cut the dough into 10–12 even slices, then place the slices on the prepared baking sheet and bake for 15 minutes until risen and golden. Transfer to a wire rack to cool.

Make the glaze as described above, then drizzle it over the cooled slices. Sprinkle with flaked almonds. These are at their best served fresh—if you like, prepare the dough the night before, refrigerate, and then slice and bake in the morning.

MAKES 10–12 SLICES

Lemon-Thyme Tea Loaf

Lemon is such a sunny, happy fruit and thyme is a herb with many wonderful qualities, both on the physical and emotional level—thyme is both healing and purifying, and it imbues us with greater courage and resilience. This simple quick bread is the perfect addition to a garden tea!

Preheat oven to 350°F and grease a medium loaf pan well.

> **2 juicy lemons**
> **1 stick butter, softened**
> **¾ cup + ¼ cup sugar**
> **2 eggs**
> **1 teaspoon vanilla extract**
> **2½ cups cake flour**
> **2 teaspoons baking powder**
> **½ teaspoon salt**
> **½ cup buttermilk**
> **2 tablespoons chopped thyme leaves**

Squeeze the juice of the lemons into a small bowl and grate the rind of one lemon finely; add to juice and set aside. In a large bowl, cream together the softened butter and ¾ cup sugar until light and fluffy, then gradually beat in the eggs, vanilla extract, and 2 teaspoons of the lemon juice.

Sift together the flour, baking powder, and salt, and stir into the butter mixture alternately with the buttermilk to form a smooth batter. Pour into the loaf pan and bake in the preheated oven for 35–40 minutes or until the cake is well risen and golden. Place on a cooling rack. Mix ¼ cup sugar with enough lemon juice to make a thick but pourable frosting. Pour over the cooled loaf and sprinkle with the finely chopped thyme leaves.

Rose and Chocolate Choux Puffs

Choux pastry is rather magical in and of itself: a sticky batter that somehow transforms itself into crisp golden puffs! (And it's really not difficult to make, either.) The filling and topping are also enhanced with the magical fragrance of roses, but please be sure to use a good quality food-grade rose essence or extract.

Preheat oven to 400°F.

Grease a large baking sheet or line it with baking paper.

Choux Pastry
- **½ cup milk**
- **½ cup water**
- **1 stick butter**
- **½ teaspoon salt**
- **1 cup flour**
- **4 eggs**

In a medium saucepan, combine the milk, water, butter, and salt, and bring to a boil. Remove from the heat and stir in the flour all at once, then return to a low heat and stir until the mixture thickens and pulls away from the sides of the pan. Leave to cool for a few minutes, then beat in the eggs, slowly and one at a time. You should end up with a soft but not sticky dough and may not need to use all the eggs.

Pipe or spoon small mounds of dough onto the baking sheet, ensuring they are at least 1½ inches apart. Again, I like to make small puffs, about 1 inch in diameter, but you can make them larger, up to 2 inches if you prefer. Bake for 15–20 minutes until the puffs are golden brown and crispy. Don't peek in the oven before they are done, as this may cause them to collapse! Turn the oven off and leave the puffs in for another 5 minutes before transferring them to a wire rack to cool.

Just before serving time, cut a small hole in the side of each puff and spoon or pipe in a little of the mousse filling. Drizzle the rose glaze over the top and serve right away.

White Chocolate and Rose Mousse

Melt 8 ounces good quality white chocolate in a bowl set over a pan of simmering water. When the chocolate is melted, remove from the heat. Whip 1 cup heavy cream, stir in 1 teaspoon each of vanilla and rose extract, and fold this into the melted chocolate. Whip 1 egg white until soft peaks form, then fold this into the prepared chocolate mixture. Chill well and use to fill the choux puffs.

Rose Glaze

Place 1 cup confectioners' sugar in a small bowl and add a few drops of rose extract and enough water to make a smooth and spreadable glaze. (A little pink food coloring can also be added at this stage.) Spoon a little of the glaze over the top of each puff just before serving.

MAKES 12–24 CHOUX PUFFS

I must be a mermaid...
I have no fear of depths and
a great fear of shallow living.

Anaïs Nin

20

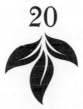

Tea with the Mermaids

*M*ermaids ... few of us haven't been entranced at some point by the myth and mystery that surrounds these beautiful creatures of the deep, living in strangely enchanted underwater realms whose blue and gold depths we can only imagine in our dreams. Apparently mermaids also have their dark side and can wreak havoc when angry or betrayed, but in general I have always liked to see them as messengers bringing us new insight, creativity, and hope from a world we cannot see or even entirely understand.

To explain this particular tea ceremony, I need to start with a personal story; it took place some years back when I was visiting the northwest coast of Scotland with my then-partner. Although it was September and supposedly a good month to visit the area, that particular year the

weather turned foul, with driving rain and winds that actually blew our tent down on our second night of camping. I was not really a happy person at that stage, and on the third day, when we visited Sandwood Bay, I was definitely in a bad mood. This is a famous and beautiful bay in the area, supposedly the haunt of mermaids who gather on the rocks and sing their ancient songs across the pale and shining sands. Unfortunately it's only reached by a long 3-mile walk through fairly inhospitable countryside, so by the time we finally reached the bay—still with rain pouring down—I was in no mood to appreciate the beauty of the place.

My partner found me a sheltered spot under a rock and said he was going to walk on a bit farther (I actually think he was a bit tired of listening to my complaints). Cold and wet, I huddled under the rock; even the picnic tea that the landlady of the guesthouse had grudgingly packed for us held no charm: stewed lukewarm tea, some rather floppy cheese and tomato sandwiches, and scones that could have been used as small missiles.

I think I must have dozed off (or perhaps the mermaids closed my eyes with a little seadust), but when I woke a few minutes later, it was to the sound of soft high beautiful voices carried on the wind. The rain had stopped, and pale sunlight lit the bay as well as the gleaming rocks just offshore—rocks that were no longer empty, for on each sat a shiny and magical creature with a long iridescent tail and pale hair that blew in the sea breezes. I don't remember how long I sat there, but I can still remember the absolute magic of that moment. I felt open, new, and blessed by all that surrounded me. The selkies (for that is the name they are traditionally known by in Scotland) are known to bring gifts of understanding, freedom, and acceptance of change on the tides of their magic, and I believe this is what they brought to me that day.

I was not happy with my life: the relationship I was in had basically run its course and we were both just going through the motions, nothing more. Other aspects of my life were out of kilter too, workwise and financially, and I was also homesick for the country where I had been born. Sitting there in that shimmering light I realized all that needed to change—and that I was the one who had to have the courage to do it. When my partner returned a little while later, I tried to tell him what I had seen, but he simply thought I had been dreaming while asleep or that perhaps I had seen seals basking on the rocks. And yes, when we returned home, I did change my life and move on, which in retrospect was a healthy choice for both of us.

I have never forgotten that day or the mermaids singing to me across the silvery sands of the bay. And since that

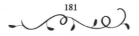

time I have also come to live at the ocean, in a place where the sea is just over the hill from my little home, and I can hear its roar and song all day and night.

Even if we are not fortunate enough to actually live beside it, the ocean is a primary source of wonder, mystery, and nourishment for our planet; it's a place of myths and mystery, of strange and transformative journeys, of both losing and finding ourselves. A friend of mine always used to say she loved being beside the sea because there she didn't have to do anything; she could simply be who she was in that moment. In many ways, that is the essence and inspiration of this book about tea, too, which is why I chose to include a special ocean-themed tea ceremony. Walking on the beach, even if it is only in our hearts, helps us remember who we are and, perhaps even more importantly, who we can still choose to be.

A few years ago, a dear friend celebrated a milestone birthday with a beach tea party, and with her permission I have included this idea here as a perfect way to enjoy tea with the mermaids. To make the table, she arranged several wooden boxes on the sand in such a way that they were fairly well-protected from both the wind and the waves; she covered the boxes in hessian (burlap) for a natural look and held the fabric in place with some large beach stones and a few beautiful pieces of driftwood.

The tea setting was simple blue-and-white cups and plates, and the table was decorated with drifts of seashells, smooth ocean pebbles, and a few delicate pieces of beach glass that we had found in the days leading up to the party. Candles consisted of white tealights set snug and safely inside glass bowls that had first been filled with sea sand. And although her birthday celebration was not specifically mermaid themed, I felt it would be entirely appropriate (and approved of) by them!

Of course, if you don't live at the ocean you might have to improvise a little, but it is possible with enough focus and intention. You might start by finding a beautiful large photo or other image of the beach or ocean to form the backdrop and intent for the gathering; you could also add shells, sand, and other ocean gifts to the table. Sea water is, as we all know, highly magical in both substance and energies, and if you can get hold of some, sprinkle it lavishly around the room where you will be holding the party, as well as lightly over yourself and the other guests. You can make a substitute for sea water by adding a little pure sea salt to a bottle of spring water and stirring well until the salt is completely dissolved.

When you are all gathered, gaze out over the ocean (or look at an ocean image) and then close your eyes. Imagine you are there, on that beautiful wild beach, with the sand

cool beneath your feet as you feel the soft ocean breezes moving through your hair and hear the haunting song of the mermaids floating towards you.

Then say the following words, either singly or together:

Mermaids, you bring us messages from the deep and mystical ocean depths. You remind us of the infinity of our earth, of the infinity of our own being. We know we are infinitely powerful and beautiful, yet sometimes we forget. Thank you for reminding us. Thank you for giving us your song and your spirit. By listening to you, we learn magic; we deepen in wisdom in all things. Thank you for giving us these gifts and for showing us how to be free. And so it is!

Mermaid Wish Bottles

A charming small gift to make for your guests at this tea celebration, wish bottles will serve as a beautiful reminder to carry ocean and mermaid wisdom in their hearts at all times. You will need small glass bottles (decorative test tubes also work well). Ensure the necks are wide enough for the shells and small pebbles you are going to add, and also that the bottles or tubes have strong corks or stoppers.

Start by placing about an inch of fine sea sand in the bottom of the bottle, then add a few tiny shells, little

pebbles, and pieces of sea glass if you can find it. Pour in enough sea water to cover the sand and shells, with a little extra room on top; the bottles or tubes should only be about two-thirds full. Place the corks or stoppers on the bottles, then tie a pretty silken or metallic cord around the neck of the bottle and add a few charms, if you like, such as shells or little mermaids. Make small labels for the bottles that say *This is a mermaid wish bottle to remind you not only of the magic of the ocean, but of the special magic you carry within you so that you may always dive and dream deep!*

Opening to Magic Tea Blend

In order to see mermaids or access the magic around or inside us, we often need a little gentle inspiration. This pretty and fragrant tea blend is ideal and will transport you to a gentle realm of enchantment as you sip.

Combine ½ cup each dried borage flowers and thyme leaves in a small bowl, then add ¼ cup dried dandelion leaves or petals. Stir in 1 teaspoon each dried fennel seeds and ground coriander, and lastly add ½ teaspoon ground ginger. Mix very well, then store the tea in a small airtight tin or jar in a cool, dark cupboard. To make the tea, place 1 teaspoonful of the blend in your cup, pour 1 cup just-boiled water over the herbs, and allow to infuse for 10 minutes. Strain and serve sweetened with a little honey.

Faerie Flower Tea

A pretty and relaxing tea blend to calm anxious thoughts and fears. All these flowers are enchanted in their restful and healing properties.

This blend is made from dried herbs and flowers, which according to faery legend you should have gathered in mid-summer under the light of a full moon. In a bowl combine 2 cups dried chamomile flowers, 1 cup dried lemon balm leaves, ½ cup dried calendula petals, and ¼ cup dried rose petals. Stir the mixture well, then store it in an airtight jar. Use 1 tablespoon of this tea mix for every cup of just-boiled water.

Jasmine Joy Iced Tea

This recipe, which I have adapted from Cerridwen Green-leaf's *Book of Kitchen Witchery*, is ideal for teas on the shore on hot and sultry summer days. It can easily be made in advance, then placed in a flask with lots of ice cubes; it can also be diluted with sparkling spring or mineral water, and you can also add a little white wine if you like.

Place 4–5 jasmine tea bags in a large jug, then add a small handful each of lemon balm and rose geranium leaves. (I prefer to use fresh herbs for this recipe, if possible.) Add a few sprigs of mint and 2 or 3 very thin slices of lemon. Pour 5–6 cups just-boiled water over the herbs and

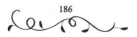

steep for 10–15 minutes. Strain the mixture, then cool it before pouring it into jugs or flasks for serving. Serve this iced tea sprinkled with extra sliced lemon or mint.

Blue Skies Tea

This simple tea blend uses beautiful blue cornflowers, which not only echo the colors of sea and sky but are linked with psychic powers and the accessing of our inner wisdom, which is ultimately the truest knowledge we can have.

You will need an oolong tea bag (such as Darjeeling), which should be placed in your cup or mug together with 1 teaspoon dried cornflower petals and ½ teaspoon dried peppermint leaves. Pour 1 cup just-boiled water over the herbs, steep for 5 minutes, strain, and serve. As you drink your tea, close your eyes and allow your intuition to take over and guide you on a new journey for your life.

Mermaid Kisses

I like to imagine these soft, sweet treats would be much-loved by mermaids. As an added bonus, they are gluten free and easy to make. I've made them with all kinds of different flavorings over the years, but this delicate lime and cardamom one is particularly delicious. The chocolate is optional; use either milk or dark chocolate, as you prefer.

187

Preheat oven to 350°F.

Line a large baking sheet with baking paper and lightly grease.

> **3 egg whites**
> **¼ teaspoon salt**
> **1 cup sugar**
> **2 cups dried, unsweetened shredded coconut**
> **½ cup ground almonds**
> **1 tablespoon finely grated lime zest**
> **½ teaspoon ground cardamom**
> **3 ounces white chocolate, chopped**

Beat the egg whites and salt together in a large grease-free bowl until soft peaks form. In another bowl, stir together the sugar, coconut, and ground almonds. Fold very gently into the egg whites—the mixture should be thick but still airy. Gently stir in the lime zest and ground cardamom.

Chill the mixture in the refrigerator for 30 minutes, then divide it into small heaps and arrange these on the baking sheet, using two spoons to make them into neater mound or cone shapes. Bake for 10–12 minutes or until just lightly golden—be careful, since they can burn easily. Cool on a wire rack. Melt the chocolate in a small heatproof bowl set over a pan of just-simmering water. (The base of the bowl must not touch the water.) When the chocolate has melted and is creamy, remove from the heat and dip the bottom of each coconut mound lightly in the chocolate. Allow to set on their sides on a large sheet of waxed paper. Best eaten fresh, which is not really a hardship!

MAKES 16–20 COCONUT MOUNDS

Champagne and Rose Cookies

Something both beautiful and a little different—an adult taste, obviously! You can use any dry or semi-sweet sparkling wine for these cookies; where I live proper champagne is just too expensive to bake with. Please remember to use good-quality culinary rose water for this recipe.

Preheat oven to 350°F.

Grease a large baking sheet well.

> **2 sticks unsalted butter, softened**
> **⅔ cup superfine sugar**
> **2 teaspoons rose water**
> **Pinch of salt**
> **2¼ cups flour, sifted**
> **¼ cup milk**

Cream the butter and sugar together well until light and fluffy, then stir in the rose water, salt, and flour; lastly, add the milk and mix with your hands to form a soft, smooth dough. Refrigerate the dough for 10 minutes, then roll out thinly on a floured board until it's no more then ⅓-inch

189

thick. Cut out suitable shapes with cookie cutters; I like flowers, hearts, and butterfly shapes. Arrange the cookies on the baking sheet and bake for 15–20 minutes or until they are a pale golden brown. Cool completely on a wire rack before frosting.

Champagne Frosting

Mix ¼ cup champagne or sparkling wine with ½ cup confectioners' sugar. The frosting should be smooth and spreadable. Spread a little frosting on each cookie, then sprinkle with a few dried or fresh rose petals. Let the frosting set before serving the cookies.

MAKES ABOUT 18 COOKIES

Salmon Mousse Pinwheels

These special and pretty sandwiches have a subtle salty flavor of the sea; you can use tinned salmon or tuna if you prefer, but the taste will be somewhat different. It's best to use either soft white or light whole wheat bread for these as the darker, heavier breads don't roll up easily. If you don't like the anise flavor of dill, try substituting finely snipped chives instead. Please note that you do need a food processor for this recipe—or, failing that, a stick blender.

> 4 ounces smoked salmon fillets (or trout)
> ½ cup full-fat cream cheese
> 2 tablespoons lemon juice

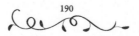

1 tablespoon finely chopped dill
Freshly ground black pepper
4 large slices fresh white bread

Place the fish, cream cheese, lemon juice, and dill in the food processor and blend to form a light, smooth mixture. Stir in a little pepper to taste.

Remove the crusts from the slices of bread and use a bottle or rolling pin to roll the bread a little thinner—no more than ¼-inch thick. Divide the mousse between the slices and spread it evenly and thinly over them. Roll up each slice tightly, then wrap it in plastic wrap and refrigerate until just before serving. Then, use a sharp serrated knife to carefully cut the rolls into pinwheels—you should get approximately six from each slice of bread. Serve garnished with extra chopped dill or chives and very thin slices of lemon.

MAKES APPROXIMATELY 24 PINWHEELS

Drink your tea
slowly and reverently, as
if it is the axis on which the
earth revolves—slowly, evenly,
without rushing toward the
future. Live the actual moment.
Only this moment is life.

Thich Nhat Hanh

21

Falling Leaves Tea

*A*utumn or fall—whatever you call it, it can sometimes seem to be a beautiful yet strange, even melancholy, season. We gather and harvest with one hand even as we must let go of summer's warmth and bounty with the other. Perhaps in this way autumn reflects the true nature of life, learning both to receive and relinquish.

The bright crunch of leaves under our feet, the changing silhouette of the trees on the horizon, and the sharpening chill of the evening air remind us that winter is just around the corner. As someone who always found autumn a difficult and sometimes painful season, I have learned (not always easily) that all things and lessons are valuable and offer us gifts if we choose to accept them; perhaps the most

valuable gift of all is to see what we have already learnt from the year and what yet remains to be discovered.

Celebrate all the harvest blessings and magic with a falling leaves tea: a perfect chance to connect with those you love at this liminal season, and perhaps to meet some people you don't yet know that well. We all have stories to tell and gifts to share, and this is the perfect time of year to remember our soul's harvest with open hands and heart.

Fall marks the threshold of the winter, a time when we need to prepare both physically and psychologically for the challenging cold months that lie ahead. One way we can do this is by preparing and storing a range of herbal tea blends that will support us in this journey; you will find some recipes and ideas for these later on in this section. It's a time to honor all we have been given thus far during the year and to celebrate that which is still to come.

If the weather permits, hold your falling leaves tea outdoors, under the bright canopy of autumn trees. Keep it simple: a wooden table and natural pottery cups, plates, and bowls. Fall is its own fabulous decorator, so simply garnish the table with sprays of berries and gathered fallen leaves, dried corn, or a ristra of dried red chiles. Gather spiky branches in a jug and tie them up with jute or twine. If you use candles, choose ones in shades of gold and green, and add a few drops of pine or sandalwood essential oil around the bottom of the wick.

To start the tea celebration, gather around the table, link hands, and one (or everyone) can say the following grace and blessing:

> *It is the end of summer, the beginning of the dark time. We have been blessed with a harvest of hope, of opportunities, of change. We have also been presented with lessons, some welcome, others not, yet they have all given our souls a place to take root, grow, and yield a good harvest. Like the leaves of the trees, we must learn now what to hold on to and what to let go of, lightly and with grace. We trust this process and our inner wisdom, and we will continue to bloom and grow even through the dark and cold that lies before us. And so it is!*

A Feather Ritual

Maybe it's just because I live in a wild place surrounded by beautiful wild birds of all kinds, but I pick up fallen feathers just about every day—and they are so incredibly magical in their variety, color, and shape. To me they are a magical representation of the fall—light, graceful, and holding the gift of flight.

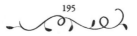

Note that collecting feathers may be illegal, depending on where you live, so it's wise to Google the rules for your particular area or country. Alternatively, make your own pretty feathers by cutting suitable shapes from light cardstock and then coloring them as desired.

A simple ritual I devised for a recent autumn tea involved the collecting of large and beautiful feathers, one for each guest. (Of course, you can make this part of the whole tea ceremony if you choose, depending on where the tea is held.) After the tea party was over and everyone had eaten and drunk their fill, I handed out the feathers, together with sheets of beautiful parchment paper I found at a local art supply store and little pots of ink (I chose sepia because I love its antique look).

I suggested that everyone write out a few things they wanted to let go of at this time, just as the trees let go of their leaves; however, since I prefer to couch things in a positive way, I also suggested that the words reflect that: for example, "I am going to explore new ways of handling conflict at home" rather than "I want to stop fighting with my partner." People could write as many as they chose, but in general it tends to be less overwhelming to have no more than three or four written down.

Dipping the feathers in the ink and writing with them took a bit of getting used to (and was not without some

muttering and grumbling), but in the end my guests were pretty good sports about it! Then we could choose to share what we had written with the group—or not—and finally everyone sprinkled their parchment with some dried rosemary needles and thyme leaves, rolled up the paper, and tied it with a beautiful ribbon or twine. The feathers we used could be added to jars or vases of natural found objects, but I often like to float them away on a nearby stream or lake. This represents, in my mind, the moving and changing nature of not only our earth, but also of ourselves. We are always evolving, always learning, and always available for earth's healing.

Moroccan Mint and Spice Tea

This is just one of my favorite tea blends, borrowed from the bright markets of Morocco, where it is served all day as both a pick-me-up and healing drink. There it is served heavily sweetened, too, but that's a matter of personal taste. Even the aroma of this tea blend is intoxicating!

Combine the following in a small bowl: 2 tablespoons dried mint, 6 crushed cardamom pods, ½ stick cinnamon broken or crushed into small pieces, 1 teaspoon dried cumin seeds, 1 tablespoon dried lemon verbena leaves, 2 tablespoons fragrant dried rose petals, and 1 tablespoon

fine dried orange zest. If you like, you can also add 1 teaspoon ground ginger. Mix all together well and store in an airtight jar or tin. Use 2 teaspoons of the mix for each cup of just-boiled water, steep, strain, and sweeten with honey or sugar.

Fall Wisdom Tea

There are many lessons we can learn from fall, one of the most powerful being to sit and wait, to let go of the drama and stress in our lives, and to allow events to unfold in their own natural time. I know this is sometimes easier said than done! Here is a simple tea blend that allows rest and calm and gives us the chance to see things in a new perspective. The honeybush tea used here is high in antioxidants and is also caffeine free.

To make one cup of this tea, place a honeybush tea bag in your cup and add 1 teaspoon each of dried valerian, fennel seeds, and caraway seeds. Pour 1 cup of just-boiled water over the herbs, steep for 10 minutes, and then strain and drink.

Negativity Begone Blend

If you are anything like me, fall can bring a sense of negativity and self-blame for things not done (or, conversely, things now done and regretted)! Sometimes we need a healthy dose of positivity to move on through these autumn days with greater self-assurance and hope. This bright and fragrant tea blend is a helpful companion on these days and should be drunk with a sense of renewed optimism and possibility.

To make this tea blend, combine ½ cup of your favorite black tea with 1 tablespoon dried lemon balm leaves, 2 teaspoons dried chamomile flowers, and 1 teaspoon dried peppermint leaves. Add a handful of crumbled dried rosehips. Mix well and store in an airtight jar. Use 1–2 teaspoons per cup to make your tea, which should be strained well before serving.

Dorset Apple Cake

This traditional English cake just seems perfect for fall, filled as it is with the warm flavor of both apples and spices. You can use any apples you choose, as long as they are lovely, fresh, and ripe. When I lived in England, various versions of this cake were popular additions to tea shop menus; I certainly sampled more than my fair share!

Preheat oven to 350°F.

Grease a deep 8-inch cake pan very well and line the base with baking paper.

2 cups cake flour, sifted

2 teaspoons baking powder

½ teaspoon each ground nutmeg, cinnamon,
    and ginger

½ teaspoon salt

½ cup raisins (optional)

1 stick unsalted butter, softened

1 cup brown sugar

2 teaspoons vanilla extract

3 eggs

2 large apples, peeled, cored, and
    chopped into small pieces

Sift the flour, baking powder, spices, salt, and optional raisins together in a small bowl and set aside. In a large bowl, cream the butter, sugar, and vanilla together until the mixture is light and creamy; beat in the eggs, one at a time. Then, add the flour mixture alternately with the chopped apples and mix well until the batter is well blended, with no streaks of flour. Use a spatula to spread the batter in the cake pan and bake for 40–50 minutes or until the cake is risen, golden brown, and a tester comes out clean. Cool in the pan for 15 minutes before turning out onto a wire rack.

This cake keeps well for a few days, stored in an airtight container. It's even nicer when served with a little heavy cream!

SERVES 10–12

Spiced Cinnamon Loaf

Cinnamon is just such a wonderful spice—and to make it even better, it's wonderfully good for us. It not only improves mood and morale but strengthens our immune system, which is a big plus as we head towards the cold winter months. This simple loaf cake is delicious on its own or with a big mug of steaming herbal or Earl Grey tea.

Preheat oven to 350°F.

Grease a medium-sized loaf pan well.

- 1¼ cups all-purpose flour
- 1½ teaspoons baking powder
- ¼ teaspoon baking soda
- 1 tablespoon ground cinnamon
- 1 stick butter, softened
- ¾ cup superfine sugar
- 2 eggs
- 2 teaspoons vanilla extract
- 1¼ cups buttermilk
- 2 tablespoons brown sugar
- ½ teaspoon ground nutmeg
- ¼ cup chopped almonds (optional)

Sift the flour, baking powder, baking soda and cinnamon together well and set aside. In a large mixing bowl, cream together the softened butter and sugar until light and fluffy, then beat in the eggs and vanilla extract. (Don't

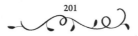

worry if the mixture looks a bit curdled; this will come right when the flour is added!) Stir in the flour mixture alternately with the buttermilk to make a soft and smooth batter. Spread in the prepared loaf pan.

Mix together the brown sugar, nutmeg and optional almonds, then sprinkle this mixture evenly over the top of the cake. Bake for 30–40 minutes or until the cake is dark golden and tests done. Cool in the tin for 15 minutes, then turn out onto a wire rack to finish cooling. This loaf will keep for a few days if wrapped airtight but tastes at its aromatic best when freshly baked!

SERVES 8–10

Little Homity Pies

These are a savory addition to an autumn tea menu, and the recipe is based on a very traditional one from England, although here I have chosen to make the pies small and bite-sized, as that just seems to work better for teatime! The potatoes in the filling are very grounding and remind us of all earth's goodness and bounty; the herbs can be varied according to personal taste, but I feel that sage or thyme are the most appropriate ones here.

You can use purchased puff or shortcrust pastry if you like and want to save time, but I would recommend giving this simple recipe a try—it's crisp and full of flavor!

Pastry

   1 cup flour
   1 cup grated cheese (such as Cheddar)
   Salt and pepper to taste
   1 stick cold unsalted butter

Combine the flour and cheese in a bowl and add salt and pepper to taste. Cut the butter into small pieces, then rub it into the flour with your fingertips until the mixture resembles coarse breadcrumbs. If it doesn't come together, gradually add a little cold water to make a soft but not sticky dough. Form into a ball and refrigerate while you make the filling.

Preheat oven to 350°F.

Grease a large baking sheet well.

   2 large potatoes
   1 onion, finely chopped
   2 tablespoons olive oil
   2 tablespoons flour
   1 egg + 1 egg yolk
   ½ cup light cream
   Freshly ground black pepper
   1 tablespoon Parmesan
   1 tablespoon chopped herbs (such as
      sage or thyme)

Peel the potatoes, chop them into small dice, and boil until just soft but not mashed. Remove from the heat, drain well, and set aside.

Fry the onion in olive oil over a low heat until soft and golden. Stir in the flour to make a paste, then add one egg and the cream and cook, gently stirring to make a smooth sauce. Add the pepper, Parmesan, and herbs, and then the cooled potatoes. Allow the filling to cool.

Roll out the chilled pastry on a floured surface to a thickness of no more than ¼ inch, then use a cookie cutter or glass to cut out circles 2½ inches in diameter. Place a tablespoon of filling in the center of each circle, then fold over carefully to form a half moon shape. Press the edges of the pies together firmly with a fork. Beat the extra egg yolk with a little water and brush this over the top of the pies— this is optional, but it gives a lovely golden-brown finish to the pastry. Bake the pies for 20–25 minutes or until the pastry is golden brown and crisp; cool on a wire rack and serve warm.

MAKES 10–12 SMALL PIES

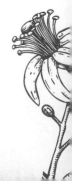

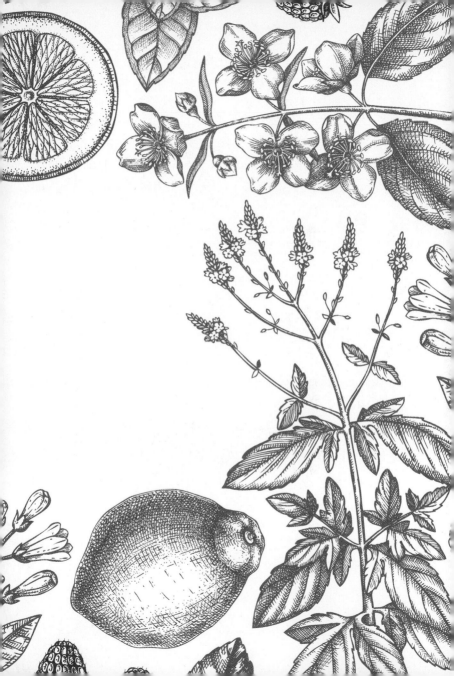

Don't wait for someone
to bring you flowers.
Plant your own garden and
decorate your own soul.

Mario Quintana

22

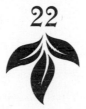

Lunar Magic Tea

*E*ven as a little girl I was fascinated by the moon. On full moon nights I would ask my mother to leave my bedroom curtains open so I could go to sleep with that clear silver light spilling across my bed; on some level I knew then that the moon holds both power and mystery over us.

And, of course, as green witches we all continue to love and celebrate Mother Moon, for we know that she is the ruler of tides, seasons, emotions, dreams, and even our physical cycles—something women are particularly aware of. Therefore, there is no better way to celebrate this mystical planet (which often seems close enough to touch!) than with a lunar magic tea, a ceremony and gathering that offers us the chance to truly honor and tap into the lunar energies all around us.

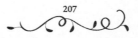

All phases of the moon carry their own magic, but it is the full moon that calls to us, as she invites us to gather and celebrate the enchanted fullness she offers to the world and to our own beings. She reminds us that we are not separate on any level but are part of the greater whole and cycle, from darkness to light and back again. This enables us to not only celebrate our own beings, but also to accept that change is a vital part of life too. A friend of mine always has a full moon tea around the time of her birthday and says it helps her remember not only where she has come from, but also where she still wishes to go. I think this is particularly valuable as we get older and sometimes feel that we are becoming invisible and losing our "value" in the eyes of society at large.

Mother Moon reminds us in the most beautiful way that although we may change as we age—which is not something to regret but rather something to appreciate and celebrate—we continue to build, nurture, and generate life in so many different ways, just as the moon continues to draw the tides of the oceans back to the shining sands.

The full moon offers the perfect occasion for a tea ritual, either with a group or on your own, depending on what you feel called to do at a particular time. However, something about the energies of this moon phase seem to call for connection and sharing, so allow yourself to be open to that when appropriate; at other times, if we are feeling emotionally stressed or uncentered, a little solitude might be more helpful and healing.

Tea Blend Ideas for Different Moon Phases

We know that each of the moon's phases brings new energies and opportunities to us; this same energy extends to all of the natural world, hence the shifting tides and growth patterns of the fields. What we are perhaps less familiar with is how we can support each of these phases within ourselves by something as simple as brewing a cup of tea.

New Moon Opens us up to new ideas and possibilities, helps us to plan for new growth with clarity and intention. Try teas made with rose, linden leaves, cardamom, bee balm, and lemon.

Waxing Moon A creative time for dreaming and putting those dreams into action, finding energy, and setting goals. Teas can include sage, rosemary, peppermint, oatstraw, and chamomile.

Full Moon The most powerful and magical phase of the moon, in which we come fully into ourselves in all our radiance, creativity, and passion. We embrace ourselves and our lives as they are. Teas to support and celebrate this time

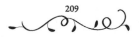

are made with hibiscus, rosemary, passionflower, valerian, and dandelion.

Waning or Dark Moon A time of retreat, rest, and renewal. We step back to look at what we have achieved, where we need to clear out and regroup, and where we need to prepare new ground for our lives. Try a tea blend that includes any of the following: lavender, willow, lemon balm, mint, nettle, or basil (particularly tulsi).

To make a beautiful moon tea ceremony, I would suggest using the following:

- Lots of silver or pale blue candles, colors which are traditionally linked to the moon

- Moonstones (if you can find them); alternatively celestite, aquamarine, or clear quartz crystals

- White tealights

- Willow branches—a tree sacred to the moon (or simply use fallen or found branches of any tree, preferably without leaves)

- Silver, white, or blue ribbons or cords

There are many goddesses (and some gods) linked with the moon in various cultures, including Isis, Hecate, Diana, and Ceridwen; you can make this ceremony specific to one of them, if you prefer, or do as I do and simply refer to Luna, or Mother Moon.

Obviously the ideal place to hold this ceremony is outside, in full light of the moon, but that may not always be possible or safe; in this case, make the room where you have the tea ritual as clear and empty as possible, and place a table as close to windows or natural light as you can. Use a pale blue tablecloth, and place a bowl filled with clear spring water (preferably lunar water; see page 28 for instructions) in the center of the table. Arrange six silver or pale blue candles around the bowl, together with some crystals of your choosing, and float a few tealights in the water.

Arrange a few willow branches in a large jug or vase and twine some ribbon or cord around and through the branches. This makes a moon tree, which ensures the continuation of blessings from the magical realms. You can also burn a little essential oil in an oil burner or diffuser before starting the ceremony; jasmine, lily of the valley, and frankincense are all appropriate fragrances.

Light the candles and gather around the table. Center and ground, drawing a few deep and healing breaths. Raise your arms and softly say the following words:

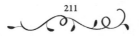

Luna, our Moon Mother, we are gathered
here on this luminous night to give thanks
for your beauty and gifts to us and our earth.
Fill us with your light and knowing as we
journey on through this earth, seeking clarity
and guidance for our path. May all gathered
here be blessed with joy and healing; may
we know our own power and use it wisely
always to bring only bright and natural
energy around us. Blessed be. And so it is!

After this is said, the candles can be blown out or not, as you prefer. It's rather magical to sit in natural moonlight sipping tea and sharing thoughts, visions, and hopes.

If you are having a tea ceremony at the new/dark moon, the energies are obviously somewhat different as this time of the month represents a shift to rest and regeneration, a necessary time in the moon's cycle, when Luna calls us to retreat into ourselves physically and emotionally. At this psychic time, allow yourself to experiment with inner journeys, divination, and spiritual dreaming. For this reason, I often think new moon tea ceremonies should be more solitary in nature or perhaps shared with just one or two close companions. Use the ceremony as given above, but afterwards blow out any candles and allow yourself to move into and through the darkness into a place of quiet renewal.

Fresh Willow Tea

This recipe is adapted with gratitude from Marysia Micrnowska's luminous book *The Witch's Herbal Apothecary*, a book which deepened my awareness of sacred earth rituals and natural medicines on every level.

When willow comes into season, harvest fresh shoots, then skin the outer bark and return it to the earth; we use the inner green bark, which should be cut into fairly small pieces and either used fresh or dried for use in the winter months.

This tea accesses deep levels of healing and awareness and helps bring us into a meditative state of lucid dreaming, which is further helped by the presence of the full moon, of which the willow is a sacred tree.

Simply infuse a handful of the chopped green inner bark pieces in a cup of just-boiled water and allow to stand for at least 20 minutes; strain and drink warm or cold.

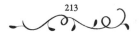

Moon Dreams Tea

This tea is both relaxing and divinatory in nature. It helps us deepen our intuitive and magical awareness, particularly when taken at the time of the full moon. Expect something enchanted to happen!

To make this blend, combine the following in a bowl: 1 cup each dried fragrant rose petals and dried skullcap, ½ cup each dried spearmint leaves and jasmine flowers (or use 2 opened jasmine tea bags), and ¼ cup dried mugwort leaves (omit the mugwort if you are pregnant). Stir the mixture lightly with your hands, then store in an airtight jar. Use a teaspoon of the mixture added to a cup of just-boiled water to make a truly insightful (and delicious) cup of tea.

Lunar Rhythms Tea

For better or sometimes worse, our physical beings and emotions are also linked to the moon and her passage through time and space; as women, in particular, we know this in the very core of our beings. Unfortunately, though, these cycles can bring with them their own issues such as PMS, pain, and irritability, but a simple herbal tea sipped at this time will gently and effectively ease these symptoms.

To make a cup of this tea, place 1 tablespoon dried raspberry leaves (known for easing cramps and regulating men-

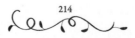

strual flow) in a cup and add 1 teaspoon dried calendula petals and ½ teaspoon dried valerian leaves. Pour 1 cup just-boiled water over the herbs, steep for 5 minutes, and serve sweetened with a little honey.

Little Lemon Balm Tarts

Milk and lemon are both sacred to the moon and used in lunar rituals of all kinds, so these delicious little tarts with a creamy herb-scented filling are ideal for serving at these magical occasions. If you prefer, you can swap out the lemon balm for lemon verbena, mint, or lavender, used in moderation! The pastry recipe makes a lot, but since the baked shells store very well in an airtight container or can even be frozen, it's great to have them on hand for all kinds of kitchen magic.

Preheat oven to 400°F.

Grease 24 small tartlet or shallow muffin pans well.

Pastry
- **1 stick unsalted butter, softened**
- **¼ cup superfine sugar**
- **1 egg**
- **1½ cups cake flour**
- **1 teaspoon baking powder**
- **Pinch of salt**

Cream the butter and sugar together until light, then beat in the egg. Sift the flour, baking powder, and salt together, then add to the butter mixture. Mix well to form a soft but manageable dough. Cover and place in the refrigerator for 30 minutes. Roll out thinly on a floured board and use a 2½-inch cookie cutter to cut out circles. Press the pastry circles into the prepared muffin or tartlet pans and bake for 10 minutes or until light golden brown and set. Cool on a wire rack before carefully lifting the pastry cases out of the tins. Store airtight once they are cool; fill just before serving time.

Custard
- **2 cups whole milk**
- **A few fresh lemon balm leaves**
- **½ cup sugar**
- **2 tablespoons butter**
- **2 tablespoons cake flour**
- **2 tablespoons cornstarch**
- **2 eggs**
- **1 tablespoon lemon juice**

Gently warm the milk and lemon balm together for 10 minutes; don't allow the milk to boil. Then strain the milk and return it to the saucepan together with the sugar and butter. Warm until the butter has melted. In a small bowl, mix the flour and cornstarch with a little water to make

a smooth paste. Separate the eggs. Beat the yolks into the flour paste, then add this to the warm milk. Cook over a medium heat, stirring continuously, until the custard is smooth and thick, then stir in the lemon juice. Remove from the stove and cool. Beat the egg whites until soft peaks form, then fold into the cooled custard mixture. Cover and keep in the refrigerator if you are not using it immediately. Just before serving, spoon a little of the custard into each pastry case and garnish with a little lemon balm leaf or some fine lemon zest.

Dreamy Moon Bars

Bar cookies are a special favorite of mine. They are versatile in that one can cut them really small for bite-sized treats or into larger bars when the occasion demands. This recipe is based on an old one, but the topping is something a bit special: cacao—dark and mysterious, sacred in its own right—makes a luscious and magical topping for these cookies; it has been used as a ceremonial drink through the ages and helps with meditation and dream work. Please, though, ensure that the cacao you buy is organic and free trade in origin.

Preheat oven to 350°F.

Grease a 9 × 13-inch baking pan well and line with baking paper.

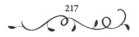

Pastry Crust

1½ cups flour

2 tablespoons sugar

1½ sticks unsalted butter, cold

Filling

¼ cup flour

1 teaspoon baking powder

½ teaspoon salt

2 eggs

¾ cup brown sugar

1 teaspoon vanilla extract

1 cup shredded coconut

½ cup pecans, chopped

To make the crust, mix the flour and sugar in a bowl; rub in the chilled butter with your fingertips until the mixture looks like large breadcrumbs. Press this mixture into the prepared baking pan to make an even layer, prick lightly with a fork, and bake in the preheated oven for about 10–15 minutes or until light golden-brown. Remove and allow to cool.

For the filling, sift together flour with baking powder and salt. In a large bowl, beat the eggs, brown sugar, and vanilla together until mixture is pale and thick, then stir in the flour mixture. Lastly, stir in the coconut and nuts, mix again, and spread the filling evenly over the prebaked crust.

Return to the oven for 25–30 minutes; the filling should be set and lightly browned. Allow the bars to cool completely in the pan.

Topping

In a small saucepan, melt together ½ cup each coconut oil and maple syrup or honey. Stir in ½ cup cacao powder, ½ teaspoon vanilla extract, and a pinch each of sea salt and ground cinnamon. Remove from the heat and allow to cool; it should be thick and creamy. Spread evenly over the cooled filling and chill in the refrigerator until firm enough to slice. Use a long knife to cut the bars into the desired size before carefully lifting them out of the baking pan.

MAKES 20–30 BARS

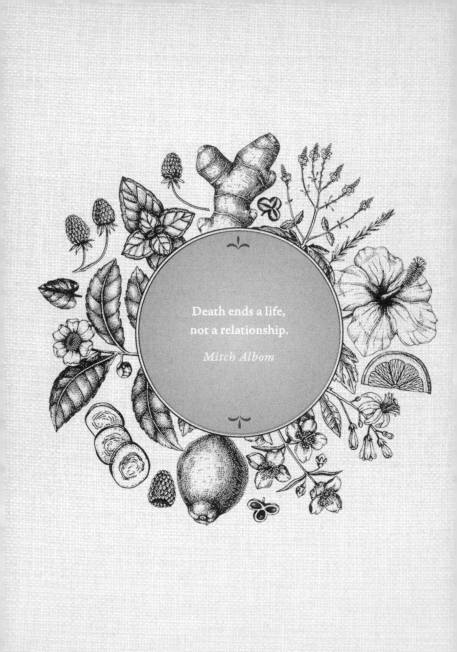

Death ends a life,
not a relationship.

Mitch Albom

23

Spirits & Memories Tea

*O*ne of the most painful and yet in its own way most beautiful realities of being human is that of loss and grief. We are going to lose people and other loved ones like pets and will have to say goodbye, often many times in our lives. And of course there are other losses too, like youth, health, beloved homes, and places we really don't want to have to leave. "This being human," as the Persian poet Rumi put it, is not always easy or for the faint of heart.

And this is something I can personally attest to, as I have lost both parents, my partner, and three close friends in the past few years. It wasn't easy, of course not, but the lessons I learned through these experiences have helped me on so many levels, and perhaps the main one is that we are not—and never—alone. Those we loved may be gone from

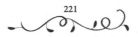

our physical sight and daily lives, but they are still woven in and through us with a silver web of connection and unseen support and hope that can both sustain and nurture us, especially on days when grief and loss seem quite insurmountable.

As the year moves through the last days of fall, we celebrate Samhain, Halloween, the Day of the Dead, and All Souls' Day; all these take place around the end of October and beginning of November, which makes this the perfect time for a Spirits and Memories tea, a way of honoring those we have lost and opening up to their messages from spirit, to the whispers and songs that are part of our history and memory. Of course this tea can be offered at other times too, particularly as a part of or following a funeral or memorial service.

I usually hold these teas at night, for the darkness seems to offer the magic and mystery the occasion demands. Candlelight is essential, preferably from black, indigo, or purple candles, which are all colors linked with death, divination, intuition, and the afterlife. The tea is usually a simple affair and should preferably include some recipes that were passed down to you by mothers or grandmothers. The sharing of recipes is one of the simplest and most powerful ways we honor and remember those who came before us.

You can decorate with traditional symbols of this season if you like—pumpkins, fall flowers and corn, little skeletons and skulls; it's up to you. I also like to add a deck of tarot or oracle cards to the table since this is the perfect time to seek the cards' wisdom and insight. Often everyone will pull a card and then quietly discuss what meaning that particular card has for them, both in terms of the theme of the tea and also as regards where they currently are in their lives and what challenges they are facing.

Tea leaf reading is another special form of divination for this type of tea occasion. You can read more about this tradition in chapter 13, The Oracle of the Leaves. There are also a number of good and insightful books on the subject.

More than some others in the book, this teatime is very much focused and centred on ritual and sometimes is best when done alone or in the company of just one or two others. Generally the sacred magic of the night reveals itself best in quiet and calm contemplation, and there are a few tea blends given below that will open us up to the hidden realms if we simply allow ourselves to relax and let go. Sit quietly, think about who you knew, who you lost, and invite them to join you now in heart and spirit. Feel their warm and comforting presence; if needed, ask for or give forgiveness so that both of you may be free from guilt or blame.

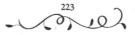

I like to spend most of this tea in darkness, with only the light of a few candles burning. This also often makes it easier for people to talk and open up about particular losses they may have experienced. When the tea has drawn to a close, I suggest everyone present stand in a circle and link hands. Say the following blessing and invocation, either singly or as a group:

> *Spirits and guides of my life, I can no longer see you, but I feel you are here with me now, in this liminal time of shadows and changes. I ask you to guide, guard, and protect me as I travel onward through my life. Be a shelter and a song of joy, and remind me I am never alone, for I feel your love around me still, and I know we will be together again in the shining lands. Blessings. Amen. And so it is and always will be!*

To me, creating small memory bags or pouches is an especially meaningful way of not only honoring those we remember at this sacred time, but of keeping the lines open between us and the spirit world on a daily basis. Each person who attends this tea ceremony can bring something specific to the person they wish to remember; photos are

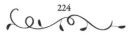

the obvious things, but I have also used letters and cards, little pieces of embroidery, old and much-loved jewellery, and more. These can be placed in a small bag or pouch to which you add a few drops of essential oil (rosemary, thyme, rose, sage, or juniper are all good) and a crystal of your choice. Ideas for crystals could include amethyst (psychic power and healing), citrine (focus and creativity), clear quartz (mental power and energy), and turquoise (protection and strength).

Other things I like to add are a charm or talisman particularly representative of the person being remembered; for my mother's memory bag, I included a tiny pewter dachshund because she absolutely loved her dogs! Perhaps you would like to include a small handwritten note or card stating what you remember and miss most about that person. Tie up the bag or pouch with a beautiful ribbon or cotton twine and hang it where you can see it every day, allowing its gentle memories and magic to heal your heart.

There are certain herbs and other plants that are particularly valuable for accessing the realms of ancestors and spirit. These include cypress, mugwort, linden, passionflower, red clover, willow, lavender, and valerian. Teas and infusions made with one or more of these plants can be very helpful for soul and heart travel of all kinds.

Lucid Dreaming Tea

This powerful tea blend will help to send you on spirit journeys to places once known and others yet to be discovered. After my mother passed away last year, I went through a painful time of not being able to feel her presence anymore; sometimes I couldn't even remember her voice. Then a friend recommended this tea, and that night I dreamt my mom and I were together again, talking happily in her flower garden, and I woke reassured of her continued presence and support in my life every day.

To make this tea blend, combine the following in a bowl: ½ cup each dried mugwort, skullcap leaves, and dried chamomile flowers (omit the mugwort if you are pregnant). Add 2 tablespoons each dried peppermint and fragrant red rose petals, then 1 tablespoon each dried passionflowers and valerian leaves. Mix well and store in a lidded jar. Use 1–2 teaspoons of this mix for a cup of tea; add 1 cup just-boiled water, steep for 5–10 minutes, then strain and drink in a quiet and reflective manner before meditating or going to bed.

Gentle Spirits Tea Blend

This idea, garnered from Cait Johnson's wonderful book *Witch in the Kitchen*, which is a constant on my cookbook shelf, is ideal for divination and connecting with spirits on

every level. The chief ingredient in this mix is mugwort, a powerful herb for accessing inner wisdom. The oatstraw is calming and makes one more open and receptive to magic. After drinking this tea, you can also use the leaves for scrying or tea leaf reading; read more about this in chapter 13. Please note this tea is not suitable for use during pregnancy.

Place 2–3 tablespoons crumbled dried mugwort leaves in a large cup and add 2 tablespoons dried oatstraw. Add ½ a cinnamon stick and pour over 1 cup just-boiled water. Steep for 15 minutes, then strain and sweeten to taste, if required, with honey or maple syrup. Sip the tea very slowly and in silence, savoring its rich taste of earth and harvest. Allow yourself to wander through different places and times in your mind, and feel the comforting presence of the spirits you have known on this earthly plane; they are still with you, bringing you their help and guidance.

Tea for Easing Grief

Grief can sometimes seem overwhelming, especially if we have recently lost someone very dear to us—we feel like our hearts are covered with a dark cloud of sadness that just won't go away, and everything is too much to deal with! If you are going through this painful time, I suggest trying this fragrant tea blend; while it obviously can't remove the emotional pain and loss, its gentle and uplifting qualities

make everything seem easier to bear as we slowly let go and relax.

Place the following in a large mug or cup: ¼ cup fresh scented geranium leaves (or you can use 2 tablespoons dried leaves, crumbled), 1 cinnamon stick, ½ teaspoon caraway seeds, 1 star anise, and a handful of fragrant dried rose petals. Pour 1 cup just-boiled water over the herbs and steep 10 minutes. Strain and sweeten to taste, if desired. Sip slowly and mindfully; allow the magic of the herbs and spices to ease and soften the pain of grief you feel.

Julia's Ancestors Tea

I consider myself very blessed to have been born and brought up in Africa, a continent so rich in history, myth, and magic. Most Africans, and certainly those in South Africa, my country, are very linked to and respectful of their ancestors and call upon their blessings and guidance in everyday activities, as well as for special occasions. Julia, who was one of my oldest and dearest friends and who had the most joyful laugh I have ever heard, often used to brew up this simple tea and sit quietly in the dark of her room "just talking to the spirit ones," as she would say. I miss her still, but when I brew this tea I know that she and I are continuing our ongoing conversation.

Very simply, brew a cup of strong rooibos tea, then stir in some finely chopped ginger, a little dried mint, and a few cloves. Stand for 5 minutes, then strain and serve; this tea is traditionally made with milk and lots of sugar—but you can omit these if you prefer!

When preparing food to serve with this tea, it's a particularly nice idea to make something that is part of your food history with the spirits you will be honoring—perhaps something they always baked for you or a recipe that has been passed down through the generations. This creates extra mojo for your tea celebration!

Guinness Cake with Midnight Frosting

This dark and luscious cake owes much of its rich flavor to the inclusion of Guinness, but you can substitute another dark milk stout if you prefer. I think it makes the perfect conclusion to tea ceremonies involving spirits and memories, for its darkness evokes the night we all have to go through in order to reach a new way of understanding and being. Plus, the Guinness echoes the Celtic spirit that is particularly powerful at this liminal time.

Preheat oven to 350°F.

Grease two 8-inch cake pans well.

2 cups cake flour

⅓ cup dark cocoa powder

1 teaspoon baking powder

½ teaspoon baking soda

Pinch of salt

1½ sticks unsalted butter, softened

1¾ cups sugar

4 eggs

1 cup Guinness

1 teaspoon vanilla extract

Sift the flour, cocoa, baking powder, baking soda, and salt together; set aside. In a large mixing bowl, cream together the butter and sugar until soft and light, then add the eggs one at a time until mixture is well blended. Add the flour mixture and Guinness alternately to the butter mixture and mix well to form a smooth batter. Stir in the vanilla extract.

Divide the batter evenly between the two cake pans and bake for 25–30 minutes or until the cakes are risen and test done. Cool in the pans for 10 minutes, then turn out on a wire rack to finish cooling completely. Make the midnight frosting and spread it generously in the middle and on top of the cooled cake. I like to garnish this with some edible fresh green leaves like mint or lemon thyme—perhaps that's just to echo the Irishness of the Guinness!

Midnight Frosting

Combine 1½ sticks unsalted softened butter, ½ cup dark cocoa, 2 cups confectioners' sugar, and 2 tablespoons Guinness in a large bowl and beat well (an electric mixer makes this job a lot easier) until the frosting is smooth and fluffy. You may need to add more confectioners' sugar if the icing is a little runny. Both the frosting and cake will keep well stored airtight in the refrigerator for a couple of days.

MAKES 8–12 SLICES OF CAKE

Rosemary and Pumpkin Muffins

Bright and bountiful, pumpkins are obviously intrinsically linked with Samhain, Halloween, and other festivals remembering those we have lost and celebrating their lives. Rosemary too is a beautiful ancient herb used in ceremonies honoring those who have passed on and can also bring much-needed comfort and courage when we are grieving. This recipe can be baked as a single loaf or as muffins, which is how I prefer it; they are best when served warm and fresh, with lots of butter and either cheese (cream or cottage) or honey. Note that you don't need to cook the pumpkin for this recipe, but please ensure you use a soft, non-stringy pumpkin and that the flesh is finely grated or shredded.

Preheat oven to 400°F. Grease 12 muffin pans well or use paper liners.

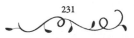

1 cup cake flour

1¼ cups polenta or yellow cornmeal

1 tablespoon baking powder

1 tablespoon honey

1¼ cups grated pumpkin

2 tablespoons finely chopped rosemary

1 cup buttermilk

2 eggs, beaten

¼ cup olive oil

2 tablespoons grated Parmesan (optional)

In a large mixing bowl, combine the flour, polenta, and baking powder, then stir in the honey, pumpkin, and rosemary. In another bowl beat the buttermilk, eggs, and oil together, then add to the flour mixture and mix well to form a batter. Divide the batter evenly between the prepared muffin pans and smooth the tops; scatter a little Parmesan on each muffin if you are using it.

Bake the muffins for 20–25 minutes or until they have risen and test done with a skewer. Cool briefly on a wire rack and then serve.

Pepper and Mushroom Mini Frittatas

These are kind of like a crustless quiche, easy to put together and deliciously savory. You can freeze them and just warm them briefly in the oven. If you prefer, the mushrooms can

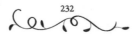

be replaced with bacon or a little cooked, chopped baby spinach.

Preheat oven to 350°F.

Grease 6–8 individual quiche pans or large muffin cups.

1 small onion, chopped

4 ounces button mushrooms, sliced thinly

1 small red pepper, seeded and chopped

Olive oil

2 eggs

1 cup cream

¼ cup cake flour

½ cup shredded Cheddar

2 tablespoons grated Parmesan

Salt and black pepper to taste

Chopped flat-leaf parsley

Fry the onion, mushrooms, and pepper in a little olive oil until soft and cooked. Cool. In a bowl, beat together the eggs, cream, flour, cheeses, and salt and pepper until mix is thick and foamy. Divide the mushroom mixture between the individual pans, then pour the egg mixture evenly in each pan. Bake for 25–30 minutes or until golden. Cool and serve warm sprinkled with chopped parsley.

MAKES 6–8 INDIVIDUAL FRITTATAS

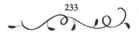

In the midst of winter,
I found there was, within
me, an invincible summer.

Albert Camus

24

A Winter Blessings & Comforts Tea

inter ... the year has grown ancient; the days are short, the nights long and frosty. Perhaps this is why many traditions and celebrations are focused around the end of the year, as a bright and joyful antidote to the cold darkness—or as a friend of mine once said, rather cynically, "Perhaps it's just a way of celebrating the fact that we managed to make it through another year!"

But the real fact is that we need to celebrate winter, just as we need to celebrate the wheel of the year in all its varied moods and colors. At this time we need to pause and reflect on the time just passed, as well as think in a meaningful and positive way about what we want to bring to the year that is just over the horizon. Winter, with its many

holidays and festivities, is an invitation to share and celebrate good things and blessings, but it is also a time for quiet thought and allowing intuition to guide us. The key is to find a balance between the two, especially in a season that can be marked with excessive busyness and stress on many levels, not to mention overconsumption and sometimes overspending.

Winter Comfort the Scandinavian Way

A few years ago the Danish lifestyle known as *hygge* (pronounced *hoo-gah*) first came onto everyone's radar, and for a while it was the topic of endless books, magazine articles, and more—so much so that I think everyone has become fairly sick of it. However, the actual ethos and reason behind the hygge lifestyle is one we should all actively embrace, especially as green witches, for it relates to the living of life with simplicity, warmth, and respect for the natural world and earth's changing seasons.

Fika is a Swedish word that refers to the practice of getting together with family, friends, workmates, or even alone for a break in the busy day—a break that usually involves something warm to drink and a little sweet bite to eat; thus it ties in perfectly with teatime tastes and rituals. Hygge is often associated with the winter months, probably because of its Scandinavian roots, and it is certainly the perfect way

to enjoy the chilly days and early darkness, with lots of candles, firelight if possible, warm clothes, and something even warmer to drink—but of course we can add a little hygge to any teatime by adding candles, gathering flowers (something as simple as a jug of daisies or dandelions), and using natural decorations like shells and wooden bowls to decorate the tea table. Place tealights in a votive or glass holder and add a few drops of essential oil: lavender for peace and harmony, rose for love and friendship, or jasmine to boost energy and increase positivity.

We all need and long to find meaning in our lives but often look for it in adventures and new experiences that are outside of the everyday routine. Teatime—and hygge—show us that it is precisely within everyday life that true magic and meaning can be found. We can make a cup of tea and sit down, either alone or with someone we care about, and find true joy in that moment. The sacred is always both with and within us.

Creating Festive Tea Magic

Green witches know this is a time of sharing and feasting together, for as human beings we have always had the instinct of sustaining ourselves and each other through the foods we grow, gather, prepare, and consume. Sadly, though, the realities of modern life often mean that the

traditions of sharing meals and celebrations have taken a back seat to fast foods and dinner deliveries. The time of Yule—of the winter solstice, the slow return to the light—is the perfect time to change this and to once again connect in love and celebration around the kitchen table.

I have always found that preparing and offering a festive tea at this time is a particularly lovely and inclusive way of celebrating without the excessive food consumption and alcohol that often goes hand in hand with other winter parties. With the teas we choose and the simple rituals we offer, we can create an atmosphere both joyful and celebratory while at the same time being a way of reconnecting to each other and to the earth that has sustained us through the year.

Creating a truly festive setting for a winter blessings tea can be as simple or ornate as you like. If you really love all the sparkle and glitter, then go for it, but to be honest I prefer keeping it as green and natural as possible, with gathered forest or garden bounty like pine cones, sprays of bright berries, and branches of natural greenery arranged in jugs or vases or draped over windows and doors. Candles—I prefer white as they echo the crisp brightness of newly fallen snow and are also indicative of the gifts of inner stillness and peace—are an indispensable part of a winter tea setting. Citrus fruit is another bright and sunny

238

gift of the winter months, so dried orange and lemon slices can be added to garlands or you can simply pile them in a wooden bowl.

I am fortunate in that I have a set of simple cream pottery teacups and plates that work well with the natural theme; I also have a wonderful teapot (bought in England many moons ago) that is white but festooned with sprays of bright holly berries. Just looking at it makes one feel festive! Obviously, you will choose your own favorites for your tea celebrations, but above all, keep it simple and joyful. As part of the tea table setting, you should also consider including some simple napkins made of either calico or red gingham, which add a further pop of color to the table. I always like to add a beautiful pot of golden organic honey to the table setting too, and not just for sweetening the tea but as a symbol of the incredible bounty we are surrounded by every day. Honey is a powerful reminder of all we have to be grateful for in our lives as we move forward into a new year with its as-yet-unknown blessings and new experiences.

When all the guests have arrived for the tea celebration, light the candles you have chosen and gather around the table, joining hands as you say the following simple Yuletide grace and benediction:

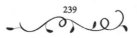

*We are gathered together at this deep and
sacred time. We honor ourselves and each other.
We honor our mother the earth, who has kept
and sustained us through this year. May we
share her gifts generously, with love, and may
we always remember we are connected, part
of the same web, part of the same mystery.
May all who share this be blessed, be safe, and
be grateful, today and always. And so it is!*

You might also want to include a simple spell or purifying ritual at the beginning of this ceremony, which I have adapted from Cait Johnson's *Witch in the Kitchen*.

Fill a small bowl with spring water and add a few teaspoons of sea salt. Stir until the salt has dissolved in the liquid, then collect a few dried bay leaves. Dip the leaves into the water and use them to sprinkle the liquid around the corners of the kitchen or room where you are holding the tea celebration; then sprinkle a little of the liquid lightly over the table too.

Softly say the following quiet blessing and invocation:

*Keep us and all within safe from harm,
keep us within the earth's green and
magic web of protection and healing,
today and always. Blessed be!*

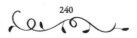

240

Votive Blessing Candles

You can make several of these—as large or small as you like, depending on the size of the glass and candles you choose. They look beautiful arranged down the center of the tea table but can also be given as small gifts for your guests to take away as a fragrant and timely reminder of this time you have all just shared.

Basically, you need glass votive holders and either small white candles or tealights. Fix the candles firmly in the base of the holder or glass. If space permits, you can arrange a few small crystals around the candle such as clear or rose quartz. Gather together some sprigs of winter greenery such as holly, pine, or fir, as well as some dried herbs: sage, rosemary, or lavender, as well as cinnamon sticks, are all possibilities. Use a piece of strong twine or decorative ribbon to tie your chosen greenery and herbs to the side of the glass, trimming them if they are too long. It's very important that none of the greenery can come into contact with the candle flame, thus creating a fire hazard.

These lights carry all sorts of magical and peaceful intentions and should be lit not only at the tea party, but also anytime we want to light our way to a new and more joyful future in the coming year.

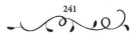

Hygge-Inspired Tea

Perfect for a late winter's afternoon, berries and spices are often added to this tea, as well as a tot of alcohol. While this one is nonalcoholic and can be served to anyone, you can add a little rum or brandy if it's really cold outside!

In a large saucepan, combine 4 cups water, 2 cups unsweetened apple, red grape, or cranberry juice, and 3 English breakfast tea bags. Add 2 orange slices, ¼ cup soft brown sugar, 1 cinnamon stick, 2 whole cloves, 1 star anise, and a pinch of grated nutmeg. Simmer over a low heat until the spices have infused and the mixture is hot. Check for seasoning, as you may need to add a little more sugar, depending on personal taste. Sieve the liquid into a heat-proof jug or bowl and then add a few additional orange slices and also a few cranberries, if you like. Serve in small glass mugs, sip, and relax.

Kindred Spirits Tea

This is the time of year when we often have the opportunity to reconnect with loved ones, friends, and family we may have drifted away from, either physically or emotionally, during the preceding twelve months. And it's important we do so since it is in our connections that we find our greatest humanness and strength, even if sometimes those self-same people drive us crazy! Sharing this simple, spicy

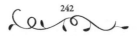

tea is a good way to reconnect and possibly break down any barriers that may have been put up, either intentionally or subconsciously.

To make this tea blend, combine 2 parts dried thyme with 1 part dried rosemary, a few cloves, 3 bay leaves, 1 star anise pod, and the dried and chopped rind of a small orange. Store in a small airtight jar or tin. To make a cup of tea, place 2 teaspoons of the mixture in a cup, add 1 cup just-boiled water, and steep for 10–15 minutes. Strain and serve. This tea tastes particularly good sweetened with honey, and you can also add a dash of rum or brandy (as a good friend of mine does) to improve the all-round positive vibes!

Fennel and Peppermint Tummy Tea

Sometimes, despite our best intentions, we tend to eat and drink a little too heartily during end-of-year festivities and celebrations and end up with tummies that feel nauseous, bloated, and painful. Making a jug of this tea ensures that you will always have a natural and effective remedy on hand; fennel has been used as a digestive since Greek and Roman times, and the ginger, chamomile, and peppermint are all soothing and relaxing for the stomach. You can store leftover tea in the refrigerator and either drink it cold or gently warm it as needed.

Place 1 tablespoon crushed fennel seeds in a jug and add 1 tablespoon dried peppermint leaves and a handful of dried chamomile flowers. Peel and thinly slice a 1-inch piece of fresh ginger and add to the herbs. Pour 2–3 cups just-boiled water over the herbs and allow to steep for 10–15 minutes. Strain and sweeten with honey.

Winter Sniffles Tea

Winter may be a magical season on many levels, but unfortunately it also often brings with it the misery of colds, flu, sore throats, and other ailments that make us less able to enjoy this time to the fullest extent. This is an old family tea recipe that can be made with dried herbs and flowers harvested from summer gardens. It holds both magic and healing in each aromatic cup.

Put 1 teaspoon each dried elderflowers, peppermint leaves, and echinacea root in a cup and add ½ teaspoon finely grated fresh ginger. Fill the cup with hot water and leave to infuse for 15 minutes. Strain, sweeten with a little honey, and add a thin slice of lemon to each cup before serving.

Blend of Abundance and Prosperity

The unfortunate truth is that the winter months and holiday season also bring with them their fair share of stress—

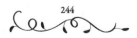

and often that stress is financial, especially in these rather difficult times. Many of us may worry about how we stretch our budget and if we are going to be able to cope with the financial demands of the new year that lies just ahead.

While I am not suggesting that drinking this tea will help you win the lottery, the herbs and spices included in it are all linked with abundance on some level, and I believe that is ultimately what we are all seeking: abundance for our lives, our futures, and our hearts.

Place 2 teaspoons green tea in your cup, then add 1 teaspoon dried lemon balm, ½ teaspoon dried thyme leaves, and a pinch of ground cinnamon. Pour 1 cup of just-boiled water over the herbs, steep for 5 minutes, and then strain and serve sweetened with a little honey, which carries its own energies of abundance and manifestation. Stir your tea clockwise three times while allowing your inner eyes to see your life as fully abundant and blessed in all things; then drink slowly and peacefully, knowing that all things ultimately come to us in their own sacred time.

Little Tea Cakes

Not really cakes at all, this very old recipe is for a soft, buttery cookie that melts in the mouth. A delightful addition to just about any tea occasion, they make a lovely and colorful winter treat. You can vary the flavor of the

fillings according to your personal taste; I have used lemon curd, dulce de leche, strawberry or apricot preserves, and a spoonful of melted chocolate (particularly nice), after which the cookies can be sprinkled with very finely chopped mint or orange zest. For the holidays they look particularly good sprinkled with extra sugar.

Preheat oven to 350°F.

Line 24 small (1-inch) muffin cups with paper liners.

1½ sticks unsalted butter, softened

⅓ cup confectioners' sugar + additional for dusting

1 teaspoon vanilla extract

2 tablespoons cornstarch

1 cup cake flour

1 teaspoon baking powder

Lemon curd, preserves, chocolate, etc.

Cream the butter, sugar, and vanilla together well, until the mixture is light and fluffy. Sift the cornstarch, flour, and baking powder together, then add to the butter mixture and mix to form a soft dough. Roll the dough into small balls and place them in the prepared and lined muffin cups. Use a wooden spoon to make an indentation in the middle of each cookie: it should be fairly deep but not go right to the bottom.

Bake the tea cakes for 15–20 minutes or until they are pale gold in color, then leave to cool for 20 minutes. Use a

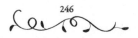

teaspoon to drop the filling of your choice into the indentation of each tea cake. Dust the cakes generously with the extra confectioners' sugar and cool completely before serving.

Nonna's Holiday Cake

This dark and flavorful fruit cake is not unlike traditional Italian panforte; it keeps well for ages, especially if you sprinkle it with a little extra brandy. It's a perfect offering for winter teas, with all the magic of fruit and honey! You can use rum or whiskey instead of brandy if you prefer, or use orange juice for an alcohol-free cake.

Preheat oven to 300°F.

Grease an 8- or 9-inch round cake pan well and line with baking paper.

> **4 ounces dates, finely chopped**
> **4 ounces raisins, chopped**
> **½ cup slivered almonds**
> **½ cup glacé cherries, chopped**
> **Chopped rind of 1 orange**
> **3 eggs**
> **⅓ cup honey**
> **1¼ cups flour**
> **½ teaspoon nutmeg**
> **¼ cup brandy**

Put the first five ingredients in a large mixing bowl, then lightly beat the eggs and add them to the mixture together with the honey, flour, and nutmeg. Mix until the batter is well combined, then stir in the brandy. Spread the mixture evenly in the prepared cake pan and bake for 1 hour or until it tests done. Cool in the tin, then store in an airtight container or wrap well in aluminum foil. Every so often, sprinkle a little more brandy over the top of the cake to keep it moist.

SERVES 8–10 WHEN CUT INTO THIN SLICES OR WEDGES

Yule Drops

These soft little cookies are redolent with spices and fruits. I have never been a big fan of the hard, crisp spice cookies traditionally made at this time of year and much prefer these! You can add whatever dried fruit and nuts you prefer, as long as the general weight is around 8 ounces. I like to add a few dried cranberries for a little burst of sharp flavor! Note that you should soak the fruit in the tea or brandy overnight, so start these the day before you plan to bake them.

Preheat oven to 325°F.

Grease a large baking sheet well.

8 ounces dried fruit such as raisins or currants
½ cup cold spiced tea or brandy

1 stick unsalted butter, softened

½ cup dark brown sugar

2 tablespoons molasses

2 eggs

2 cups cake flour

⅛ teaspoon baking soda

1 teaspoon ground cinnamon

1 teaspoon ground nutmeg

½ teaspoon ground ginger

½ cup chopped nuts (optional)

Soak the fruit in the liquid, preferably overnight, then drain and reserve the liquid.

In a large bowl, beat together the butter, sugar, and molasses until the mixture is light and fluffy. Beat in the eggs one at a time. Sift the flour with the baking soda and spices and stir into the butter mixture. Then add the fruit and the liquid it soaked in; if the batter is very stiff, stir in a few tablespoons of milk. Lastly, add the chopped nuts if you are using them.

Drop spoonfuls of the batter onto the prepared baking sheet, leaving a little space between the cookies, and bake for 15–20 minutes or until light golden-brown. Cool on a wire rack and store in an airtight container.

MAKES 20–30 COOKIES

You must live in the present,
launch yourself on every wave,
find your eternity in each moment.

Henry David Thoreau

25

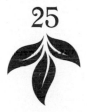

Herbs, Spices, Plants & Flowers Used for Teas

This chapter serves as a quick reference for tea making and magic, and it includes basic information about plants used for tea-making purposes: this includes their general and health uses, magical and spiritual correspondences, and contraindications for use, if any. Please note this is simply intended as a guide for the more generally known and available plants used for tea purposes, which can usually be cultivated or purchased in many areas of the world. There are, of course, many more herbs and teas specific to certain countries and cultures, but for this little book I have chosen to keep it fairly simple and accessible. You can use this list as a stepping stone for developing your own unique teas and blends, according to personal need and preferences—this is the ultimate goal and

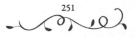

experience of being a green witch, as we travel on our own journey of discovery and magic.

Please remember that, as far as possible, you should only use herbs (fresh or dried) that you have either grown yourself or purchased from a reputable source such as a natural foods store or a farmers market. This avoids the likelihood of your herbs being tainted by pesticides and the like. I buy my dried herbs from a very reputable food store group that not only insists on all their herbs being grown organically, but also does not use GMO seeds or irradiation on their products.

For foraging and gathering herbs and other plants in the wild, please see the notes starting on page 44.

In general, the plants in this list are safe to use for home medicinal and ritual purposes. Each listing includes any contraindications or general precautions for using these plants. However, there are some plants that are highly toxic and should not be used at all for teas or any other herbal purposes, although I can't imagine anyone would try to! The point is that some plants look and smell exquisite (lilies of the valley and moonflowers, for example) but are really poisonous!

A brief list of these toxic plants that most of us might encounter at some point includes azaleas, baby's breath, clematis, crocus, daffodils, datura, foxglove, hyacinth, hydrangea, iris, lily of the valley, lobelia, moonflower, morning glory, oleander (beautiful but deadly!), plumbago, poinsettia, sweet pea, tomato (leaves), Virginia creeper, wisteria, and yew.

Two herbs that raise some questions are rue and pennyroyal. I have included rue in this section as it does have some medicinal value, but there are many modern herbalists who choose not to use this herb at all, and if you have any doubts, it's best to err on the side of caution. Pennyroyal, a member of the mint family, was extensively used at one stage, but this is no longer advised by herbalists.

Anise Hyssop (*Agastache foeniculum*)

This pretty and sweetly fragrant herb is part of the mint family, and its delightfully fluffy long mauve flowers look charming in a herb garden; it can also be grown in a medium pot or other container. Anise hyssop is a cleansing and purifying herb and was used as such by some Native American tribes for sacred rituals and ceremonies. It's a gently uplifting herb with a mild yet delicious aniseed flavor, and used in tea will help lift the spirit and ease low, sad feelings. Medicinally it can be used for coughs, colds, and to encourage sweating. Create herbal syrups with the leaves and use them for teas, baking, and desserts.

Apple (*Pyrus* spp.)

A fruit that needs no introduction, the apple has been a part of history, legend, and magic since time began (or almost!)—every part of the fruit can be used, and that holds true of herbal teas too. Fresh apple juice can be added to all sorts of different tea blends or to jugs of iced tea for a different flavor profile. Thinly sliced apples, either fresh or dried, can be floated in cups of herbal tea.

Apples have so many different magical associations—they are linked to the dead and the afterlife, so are excellent to use for teas at Samhain, Halloween, or any ceremonies honoring souls that have passed into the light. Eating apples is said to open portals into unseen realms and help us gain new knowledge and insight; they are also indicated for healing, love spells of all kinds, and creating greater abundance in our lives, on whatever plane. Pears also have magical associations of love, passion, and prosperity, and can often be used instead of apples in tea blends—either in the form of pure pear juice or slices of fresh pear.

Ashwagandha (*Withania somnifera*)

The dried root of this plant, long a feature of Chinese medicine, can be used in teas and infusions. It's an adaptogen that helps return the body to a state of well-being and balance. Use this plant when you want to feel less anxious or have better concentration and increased energy.

Basil (*Basilicum* spp.)

This is one of the most versatile and useful herbs, but for herbal tea purposes tulsi, or holy basil, is the one most often recommended. It's sacred to Hindu belief and is considered to be the holiest of all herbs. However, there are more than sixty different species of this beautiful plant, with flavors ranging from lemon to liquorice, and most can be used for tea purposes. Because it grows easily in pots and window boxes, it's also an extremely useful addition to kitchen or windowsill gardens. Holy basil tea is renowned for helping remove spiritual and emotional negativity, creating more healthy energy in body and mind, and helping balance the chakras, the seven energy centers of the body. All basil is uplifting and good for depression or fatigue.

It's an anti-inflammatory herb, and a cup of basil tea daily can help with arthritis and similar conditions; as an adaptogen, it helps the body deal with stress and toxins, and it encourages better sleep. It's good for digestive issues and prevents vomiting and nausea. However, it's also a powerful herb and should be used with caution if you have liver problems or are taking medication for diabetes, hypertension, or blood-clotting problems. During pregnancy basil should be used with care and in very limited quantities.

Bay Tree (*Laurus nobilis*)

This beautiful tree is native to the Mediterranean and has a long and noble lineage, as its name suggests. In Greek and Roman times, it was used in sacred temple rituals, and wreaths of laurel were used to crown great warriors and heroes. It's a fairly large tree but can be grown in a pot if necessary, trimmed regularly to prevent it from becoming top heavy.

Bay leaves can be used fresh or dried (the fresh are much stronger). These leaves are an indispensable part of many traditional recipes, particularly in France and Greece.

Medicinally, bay is a protective and warming herb that can help ease headaches and soothe the pain of aching limbs and joints. The leaves can cause skin irritations if applied topically, and bay should be used in limited amounts during pregnancy.

Bay leaves are said to increase psychic and prophetic powers and visions; use them in teas when you need protection, healing, strength, and increased wisdom in any sphere of life.

Bergamot (*Monarda didyma*)

Also known as bee balm, this herb is native to North America and was originally used as a healing and restorative tea by the Oswego Nation; it's akin to the bergamot orange leaves (used in Earl Grey tea) in flavor. In fact, a

fresh leaf of bee balm can be added to a cup of black tea to mimic the taste of Earl Grey. It can be used fresh or dried as needed.

Blackberry (*Rubus fruticosus*)

Such a delicious and familiar fruit-bearing bush—both leaves and fruit can be used for tea purposes. An intensely magical plant, the blackberry is associated with protection (probably because of its spikes!) as well as prosperity and fertility. Blackberries are a favored fruit in the faerie world, so if you are trying to see the fae, you would do well to make iced tea using a few blackberry leaves or bake some berries into a pie or scones.

On a more serious note, blackberry leaf infusions can be drunk to ease stomach upsets or cystitis; they are a general tonic and diuretic. However, just like raspberries, blackberries can be a uterine stimulant so should be avoided in the first months of pregnancy.

Sliced, the fruit makes an attractive addition to iced teas. You can also dry the fruit—something of a messy business—then chop them finely and add them to tea blends.

Borage (*Borago officinalis*)

This pretty plant is also known as starflower, a name that is easily explained by the shape of its delicate blue-violet flowers. Borage is the ultimate "happy herb" and has

257

been employed by herbalists and natural healers for centuries for its uplifting properties that help both body and spirit. Bees love borage too and it makes a wonderful companion plant, particularly for strawberries and tomatoes.

Borage tea helps alleviate the symptoms of coughs, colds, and fevers, as it is both cooling and cleansing on the body as a whole. With its soothing and calming properties, it's also particularly useful in alleviating depression, anxiety, or stress-related conditions of all kinds.

The flowers can be used fresh or dried and can also be added to a jug of iced tea.

Buchu (*Barosma betulina*)

This is a South African plant that originated in the Cape, where it was used by the Khoi San people both as medicine and for its pleasant blackcurrant fragrance. It makes a very palatable addition to the herbal tea cabinet, and as a warming and stimulating herb is useful for toning various parts of the body, in particular the kidneys and urinary system.

Unless we happen to live in the Cape Province, it's unlikely that we will be able to access fresh buchu leaves so we will have to make do with dried, which are actually quite a lot stronger and more pungent. In fact, buchu is an extremely powerful herb that should be used in moderation—no more than 1 teaspoon per cup of tea. (There's an old recipe that involves steeping buchu leaves in red wine with cloves, spices, and sugar, and then taking a cup of this to relieve the aching misery of colds, flu, and fever—not for the fainthearted!) This herb should always be used in moderation and avoided during pregnancy or when breastfeeding.

Calendula (*Calendula officinalis*)

An herb that's been in use since ancient Egyptian times, calendula is a member of the daisy family, and its bright flowers bring extra sunshine to any garden! Both leaves and flowers can be used for tea and other herbal purposes; pick and use fresh when in bloom, then dry some for future use. It has many medicinal uses, but in particular it's an anti-inflammatory and is great for relieving digestive prob lems, infections (particularly those of the skin), menstrual cramps, menopause symptoms, and more.

On the emotional level, calendula can help us resolve unhelpful or toxic beliefs so we can move forward with greater energy and a more positive outlook. This bright and sunny plant encourages a more childlike and joyful approach to our lives and any problems we may be currently experiencing. Calendula is a wonderfully simple and accessible plant ally and should be part of every herbal tea garden. Please note that calendula should not be taken internally when pregnant or breastfeeding.

California Poppy (*Eschscholzia californica*)

This bright and beautiful plant, native to North America, has been used by Native Americans for centuries, chiefly for its relaxant and calming qualities. (It's related to the opium poppy but lacks the hallucinogenic effect!) The poppies grow easily in most garden conditions (including in pots) and will add a vibrant touch of color and warmth to any garden—additionally, they attract bees, which can only be a good thing.

Leaves, flowers, and stems can be harvested and used fresh or dried for later. Teas made with poppy have a calming and mildly sedative effect, good for times of nervous stress, anxiety, or when you can't sleep. The plant is also a mild pain reliever, especially for headaches and toothaches.

Caraway (*Carum carvi*)

To me caraway is always somehow associated with old-fashioned Victorian teas, when caraway cake was a standard item on the tea table—but this spice has a much longer history: seeds have been found in archaeological sites dating back 5,000 years. This plant was revered for its strong healing powers, and although these days we tend to think only of using caraway seeds, in actual fact the leaves, roots, and young flowers are also used for culinary and healing purposes.

Lightly crushed caraway seeds, with their subtle and haunting flavor, can be used for teas and infusions, and are helpful for indigestion, flatulence, and menstrual cramping and pain. The ground or crushed seeds can also be added to breads, cakes, and cookies. Caraway is reputed to have the power to attract love or keep lovers from straying and is also a generally protective herb in the home. Don't use caraway medicinally if you are pregnant or breastfeeding.

Cardamom (*Elettaria cardamomum*)

With its warm and evocative flavor and fragrance, this spice has been around since ancient times and was used by the Egyptians, Greeks, and Romans before it made its way into Europe along the fabled caravan routes. It's much used throughout Africa and the Middle East, both in the kitchen and as a medicinal spice.

These fragrant seeds are an excellent digestive remedy, help with mouth and gum problems (including bad breath), and also make a mild but effective painkiller, particularly for toothaches and sore throats. On the emotional level, cardamom will increase feelings of love and desire, so it is ideal when you want to bring a little more romance into your life! More than that, though, this spice is linked with friendship and connection of all kinds and opens us up to receiving and giving human warmth and grace.

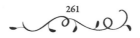

It's possible to buy cardamom already ground, but in general I prefer to buy the whole seeds; store them in an airtight glass jar in a cool dark place and use them as they are or crush as many as you need in a mortar and pestle. Please note that it's best to avoid large amounts of cardamom if you are pregnant or breastfeeding.

Catnip (*Nepeta cataria*)

Also known as catmint, this herb is aptly named as cats go wild for its fragrance! It's actually part of the large mint family and grows happily in containers; the leaves, with their lemon-mint flavor, can be used fresh or dried and added to herbal tea mixtures.

Catnip is helpful for colds, flu, and other feverish conditions, as well as easing digestive issues and upset stomachs. It's a calming herb and as such can be used as a mild sedative in difficult or stressful situations.

German Chamomile (*Matricaria recutita*)
Roman Chamomile (*Anthemis nobilis*)

These plants, very similar in their uses, are both essential in any herbal tea repertoire. A dainty and sweetly scented plant, chamomile helps bring us back to "the sunny side of the street" by removing blocks and challenges, whether these come from our own thinking or as the result of outside negative influences. Chamomile tea is probably best

known for helping us get a good and peaceful night's sleep by easing nighttime anxiety and fears that may keep us awake in the wee small hours of the morning, staring into the darkness. And it works very well for children, too.

Chamomile works both medicinally and magically as this plant is traditionally renowned for supporting life energies on multiple levels. It's an anti-inflammatory and analgesic ideal for treating digestive issues, skin problems, urinary tract infections, and menstrual problems, including PMS and cramps. On the spiritual level, chamomile helps us deal with anger and the feeling of being disconnected from life, and it's particularly good when we are going through the pain of grief and loss.

Chervil (*Anthriscus cerefolium*)

Another ancient herb dating back to Roman times, this is probably not a particularly well-known herb these days, which is a pity because it has many medicinal uses as well as being used in French cuisine as part of the traditional fines herbes. As such, the delicate leaves, which have a parsley and aniseed flavor, are used in salads, soups, sauces, and fish dishes.

A tea made of an infusion of the fresh green leaves may be drunk to improve sluggish digestion and stomach complaints; it also improves circulation and chronic catarrh.

Chickweed (*Stellaria media*)

An instantly recognizable annual that grows all over the world, with little star-shaped white flowers that grow on long and trailing branches. For some people this plant is nothing more than a garden weed to be eradicated as ruthlessly as possible, while for others it is both edible and medicinally valuable.

Chickweed is full of vitamins and minerals, and the fresh leaves can be eaten in salads or cooked as a vegetable. The leaves, either fresh or dried, can also be infused into teas; the herb is particularly renowned for helping regulate kidney function and control water retention in the body. In folk medicine it was reputed to be an aid to fertility and also a herb for cooling anger and resentment, thereby improving relationships.

Cinnamon (*Cinnamomum verum*)

Probably one of the best known and most useful of all the spices. With its familiar warm scent and flavor, cinnamon is versatile and can be used for culinary, medicinal, and cosmetic purposes. Cinnamon is full of solar energy, and this gives the spice its warming, energising, and healing properties. Cinnamon tea—either on its own or added to other tea blends—is wonderful when used in rituals of all kinds, especially those involving spirit connection, divination, and healing. It's an ancient remedy for stom-

264

ach problems, including nausea and diarrhoea, and is also helpful for winter ailments such as coughs, colds, and sinus infections. It reduces high blood pressure, a major cause of heart disease and strokes. However, it should not be used in large quantities by diabetics, as it lowers blood sugar levels. People with liver problems, pregnant and breastfeeding women, and very young children should use cinnamon in moderation.

Cloves (*Syzygium aromaticum*)

The clove seeds that most of us are familiar with are the dried flower buds of this tree; they pack a powerful punch and should always be used with discretion as their beautiful aroma can quickly take over and become overwhelming! A tea made with dried cloves can help with muscular aches and pains and is also helpful for vomiting and gastric cramping. Cloves are also an ancient remedy for toothache. When we are going through stressful situations that are leaving us confused and unable to concentrate, cloves stimulate both mind and spirit and help improve memory. Do not take for long periods of time. The tea is best avoided during pregnancy and when breastfeeding.

Clover (*Trifolium pratense*)

Please note that this refers to red clover although white clover (*Trifolium repens*) is also widely used; these plants

(sometimes unfortunately regarded as noxious weeds) have a long and illustrious history that dates back to the times of the ancient Druids. They were believed to be the bearers of luck and prosperity, and a cup of clover tea was an old and trusted country remedy for all kinds of ailments, from coughs and arthritis to liver problems and eczema. Both flowers and leaves, either fresh or dried, can be used for teas and infusions; the flowers can also be chopped and added to iced teas.

Comfrey (*Symphytum officinale*)

This perennial plant with its large green leaves is native to Europe, much of North America, and Siberia. It is an ancient folk remedy as well as being sacred to all manner of green witch rituals. Comfrey was known as "knitbone" in days gone by for its ability to heal all kinds of injuries, as well as burns and rashes. (It's still used for this but should not be applied to very deep wounds as it can heal the surface of a wound very quickly while there is still infection trapped in deeper layers of skin tissue.) It's also an expectorant for coughs and other ailments of the respiratory system, as well as being helpful for sore and painful tummies and acid reflux disease.

Mostly, however, comfrey can be used on the emotional level for helping us through difficult times of loss and

trauma as we seek new ways of being in the world and draw on deep reserves within our hearts and souls. Comfrey is a powerful ally in this journey and process.

Tea can be made with the leaves or added to blends for these purposes; the leaves should preferably be used while quite young since older leaves may contain higher levels of an alkaloid with potentially harmful effects on the liver. For this reason, the herb is best avoided if you have liver problems and also should be used carefully if you are pregnant; in any event, do not consume comfrey for more than a few days at a time.

Coriander/Cilantro (*Coriandrum sativum*)

Love or hate it, coriander (more generally known as cilantro in North America) is a powerful and ancient herb; Sanskrit documents dating back 7,000 years record its cultivation and use. All parts of the plant are edible—leaves, roots, stems, and seeds; the green parts are an essential part of the cuisines of India, Asia, North Africa, and Mexico, and the seeds make a wonderful addition to pickles, chutneys, and curry sauces.

Coriander (green parts) is a diuretic and antibacterial herb, making it useful for cleansing and calming the system. It's warming and can help relieve pain, especially headaches, neuralgia, and the discomfort of arthritis or rheumatism. The leaves and other green parts of this plant are best

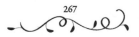

used fresh, as they lose much of their aroma and distinctive taste when dried. However, the seeds can be stored whole in small airtight jars or tins and ground as needed; roasting them before grinding is traditionally done to increase the wonderful flavor and aroma of these spicy little wonders.

Cornflower (*Centaurea cyanus*)

This pretty plant with its fluffy blue flowers is not just a lovely addition to the garden, but also has a long history of magical and medicinal use. The flowers were believed to repel evil and protect against harmful forces of all kinds, and have been used in traditional and Pagan rituals for centuries.

Medically an infusion of the flowers has been used as an eyewash (and was also reputed to open the third eye); the flowers can be added to teas and are a general tonic and stimulant for the system. Dried flowers have a delicate, spicy flavor and can also be added to salads, cold beverages, and cakes.

Cumin (*Cuminum cyminum*)

This delightful, warm spice is very familiar to those of us who love curries and other traditional dishes from India, the Middle East, and Mexico, but it also has a far wider range of uses. The whole seeds can be added to tea blends (in moderation); although ground cumin is much used in

cooking, I don't personally use it in teas as I find it often makes an unpalatable paste in the mixture. In India it's used as a medicinal remedy for all types of digestive issues, like flatulence and diarrhoea, but this spice also has ancient magical powers of protection and the removal of malevolent forces. It's also credited with improving lust and passion, so it might be a good addition to teas shared with a significant other!

Dandelion (*Taraxacum officinale)*

What can one say about this tough, tenacious, beautiful little plant that offers us its bright flowers even in the most challenging of circumstances? Perhaps that's a good lesson for life in general! Some regard dandelion as both a nuisance and invasive weed, but for the herbalist dandelion is an incredibly useful plant that has been used for centuries on both the medicinal and emotional level.

Dandelion is an alterative: it detoxifies and cleanses the body. Teas and infusions, which can be made from the leaves, flowers, or stems of the plant, help treat liver and gallbladder problems, joint pain, skin issues, fevers, urinary infections, and more. Emotionally, dandelion reminds us to stand tall and that we have value and something special to offer the world—a valuable gift for times when we are feeling low or lacking in self-esteem. Plus, a jar of the dried

flower heads in the herbal tea pantry just reminds us of summer magic, both within and without.

Dandelion does have diuretic properties, so be aware that it can reduce the efficacy of any medication you take.

Dill (*Anethum graveolens*)

A delicate herb with feathery leaves often used in cooking, particularly when preparing egg and fish dishes or sprinkled over salads. Part of the same family as fennel, dill shares some of its anise flavor and can be quite strong and pungent, so should be used in moderation. Dill seeds are the strongest part of the plant and can be used for both cooking and medicinal purposes, as can the pretty little flowers. Dill is an excellent digestive herb and remedy for stomach complaints; it's also good for bad breath that might stem from digestive issues. It eases fevers and helps strengthen nails, hair, and bones.

Magically, dill helps protect us from bad or destructive forces and hexes of all kinds. Use it in teas when you want to encourage honesty in relationships or for fertility issues. This gentle herb is generally safe for most people and can be used for children too.

Echinacea (*Echinacea purpurea*)

Native Americans have used this plant, indigenous to the North American continent, for a myriad number of

healing and other purposes for centuries, but its popularity has spread worldwide in recent times. It's a visually stunning prairie plant with distinctive purple petals surrounding a golden cone. The number of this herb's healing properties are truly amazing, but echinacea is primarily a natural antibiotic and immune stimulator that encourages the body's natural system to remove viruses and bacteria and bring about rapid and effective healing. It's also useful for fungal infections, mouth ulcers, and general cold/flu/sinus issues.

Teas can be made with fresh leaves, flowers, or roots; these can also be dried and stored in an airtight jar. Please note that this tea should not be used continuously, but rather used for up to fourteen days before taking a break.

Elderflower (*Sambucus nigra*)

Used all over the world for centuries, this ancient tree is seen as possessing powerful medicine and magic; it was revered by both the Celts and Druids, and is associated with many ancient legends as well as being known for protecting from negative energy, evil, and bad luck. It's also traditionally associated with death and the afterlife and was often used during funeral rites.

All parts of the tree are used as both remedy and enchantment. The berries must be cooked before use and the leaves are poisonous if taken internally. However, it's

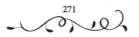

the beautifully delicate white sprays of flowers that the elder is most known for—flowers that can be made into a tea that is helpful in treating colds, allergies, sinusitis, and fevers. The flowers also lend their magic sweetness to herbal syrups and cordials that can be added to teas (both hot and iced), desserts, and baked goods.

The elder tree reflects the seasonal changes in the garden so wonderfully—from the abundance of spring blossoms to the colors of late summer berries to the bare-bones clarity of the winter months. So, too, can we learn from this magical tree to accept the cycles of our own lives and work with them with awareness to find new wisdom and knowledge.

Eucalyptus (*Eucalyptus globulus*)

Few of us are not familiar with the distinctive, fresh, and antiseptic aroma of eucalyptus leaves, which are widely used for a number of commercial medications, in particular those for coughs and colds as well as remedies for aching joints and sore muscles. The leaves can be used fresh or dried in herbal teas and infusions; however, they should be used with caution and in limited quantities since they are quite strong and high in volatile oils. Apart from easing winter illness miseries, eucalyptus helps us focus and improves concentration, especially when we are suffering from burnout or mental exhaustion.

Evening Primrose (*Oenothera biennis*)

A tall and beautiful plant with bright yellow flowers, for centuries evening primrose was mostly used for culinary purposes until research done in the 1980s revealed the healing powers it contained, particularly in the seeds. (However, all parts of the plant can be used: leaves, flowers, stems, and roots.) Evening primrose oil contains gamma-linolenic acid (GLA), an essential fatty acid that the human body cannot produce by itself. The medicinal value of evening primrose covers many different conditions, ranging from asthma to skin problems and circulatory issues to menopause. However, it is as an antidepressant and stress reliever that this herb really stands out—with some cautionary notes. A tea or infusion can be made with leaves and flowers but should be consumed with some care, particularly if you are epileptic or on antipsychotic medication of any sort. Don't use evening primrose if you are pregnant or breastfeeding.

Fennel (*Foeniculum vulgare*)

An ancient herb mentioned in Greek mythology and regarded as a gift from the gods, a way to banish malevolent spirits and encourage hope and positive energy. A tea with fennel seeds is great for ceremonies of purification and cleansing or simply when one is feeling down, lethargic, or lacking in creativity on any level. Medicinally, it's anti-inflammatory and can be used for stomach issues or to

273

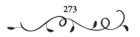

detoxify and cleanse the body. As it is also a uterine stimulant, it should be avoided during pregnancy, but its mild oestrogenic effect can be helpful to ease the symptoms of menopause.

Fenugreek (*Trigonella foenum-graecum*)

These aromatic seeds have been used as a culinary spice for centuries, particularly in curry dishes, breads, and drinks, but fenugreek is a powerful little magician in its own right, for not only does it banish negative forces and diseases, but it helps increase prosperity and good health on all levels. If we feel we are "losing the plot" as regards our lives and what direction to move in, adding a few fenugreek seeds to our herbal teas will help us regain both clarity and energy.

Tea made with fenugreek seeds is helpful for sore, painful throats and also may help relieve some of the symptoms of menopause, as the seeds contain chemicals similar to female oestrogen. Fenugreek should be avoided in pregnancy and should not be taken for long periods at a time as it can cause stomach upsets. Large amounts of this spice can alter blood sugar levels, so use with care if you are diabetic.

Feverfew (*Chrysanthemum parthenium*)

Also known as wild chamomile, this plant looks similar but has more leaflike foliage. It's also a lot more pungent and sharper in flavor; the fresh or dried leaves and flowers can be used in teas and infusions. This is a tonic herb that also helps with headaches and migraines, indigestion, menstrual complaints, and fevers. Feverfew was reputed to help remove hexes and other toxic energies and protect against illness of all kinds.

Fir (*Abies* spp.)

There are dozens of members of this conifer family, all originally native to the Northern Hemisphere; essential oil is made from its sticky resins and has an instantly recognizable fragrance. A tea made from the flat needles of fir trees can help with health issues like headaches, colds, sore throats, and other respiratory ailments. Emotionally, the plant offers uplifting and relaxing energies and is believed to help us access higher, clearer visions for our lives.

Geranium (*Pelargonium* spp.)

Please note that this only refers to the scented variety of geranium, which is indigenous to South Africa; there are many different fragrances of this plant, but the ones that are probably most useful in a herbal tea repertoire are *Pelargonium graveolens* (rose-scented) and *Pelargonium tomentosum* (peppermint). Easy to grow, these plants also do well in containers.

Used singly or mixed with other herbs and flowers, the leaves and flowers of the plant can be used, and the leaves also dry fairly successfully, although I have found they lose some of their distinct fragrance within a few months. These herbs all have a similar relaxing, calming, and antidepressant effect, and they are excellent for helping with insomnia, anxiety, and stress-related digestive problems. It's also a mild painkiller and is helpful for menopausal issues, but as these plants have a mild hormonal effect, they are best avoided during pregnancy. However, this plant can be used for children in moderate amounts, especially for kids who are shy, afraid, or struggling with issues at school or home.

Ginger (*Zingiber officinale*)

Probably one of the most widely recognised and loved spices throughout the world, ginger is another powerful magnet for magic; it purifies and increases spiritual energies both before and during rituals and ceremonies and has been used for this purpose down the centuries. It's also a revitalizing spice—in the bedroom too—and was even mentioned in the Kama Sutra; it's also an anti-inflammatory agent, so ginger tea can be helpful for arthritis and other painful joint conditions. The warming magic of ginger can ease the misery of colds and flu as it stimulates circulation and helps the body get rid of toxins. Ginger is generally safe when used in moderate amounts, but large quantities of ginger tea are best avoided if you have gallstones or are diabetic, as the spice can lower blood sugar levels.

Ginkgo (*Ginkgo biloba*)

This ancient Asian tree dates back to prehistoric times and can live for a thousand years or more. Sacred to Buddhists and extensively used in Chinese medicine, the tree was in danger of becoming extinct at one point but has undergone a resurgence in recent years, with the ginkgo biloba leaf being credited with helping to ease depression, memory loss, and ADHD. Many people swear by this plant as a way of clearing and clarifying thought processes, particularly in times of stress and anxiety. Leaves and seeds are used, but in general it's the dried leaves that are added to teas and tinctures. Some herbalists recommend that this plant is only used under medical supervision and in limited quantities.

Goldenrod (*Solidago virgaurea*)

A well-known healing herb since medieval times (it was a favorite of Culpeper, the most famous herbalist of his day, who believed it was the superior herb for treating all kinds of ailments), this bright yellow plant was also used by Native Americans for complaints such as kidney stones

and urinary tract infections, back pain, allergies, hayfever, and as a calmative in stressful stituations.

Tea can be made from fresh or dried flowers and leaves and has a fresh, aromatic taste; it can also be added to teas that are slightly less pleasant to the palate to make them more palatable.

Gotu Kola (*Centella asiatica)*

The Latin name of this low-growing herb indicates its Asian origins: also known as pennywort, it has long been used in Chinese medicine, where it was purported to bring about both longevity and stamina of body and mind. It is a remarkable herb that speeds up the healing processes, improves circulation, and detoxifies the body, while also sharpening up focus and concentration. It was often used during meditation or for spiritual rituals.

Drinking this tea will balance and improve mood and strengthen your nervous system, especially in times of anxiety or stress. However, this herb should be used in moderation, as excessive use can cause headaches; it should also be avoided if you are pregnant, breastfeeding, are taking sedatives, or have thyroid problems.

Hawthorn (*Crataegus* spp.*)*

This plant genus includes both trees and shrubs; they all have flowers and small rosy-colored fruit. These, as well as the leaves, are edible and have been used for medicinal purposes for centuries. In ancient Greece hawthorn was given as a heart medicine and is still used for that purpose today. Chinese medicine also makes extensive use of hawthorn, particularly for digestive complaints.

Hawthorn was a sacred tree in both Celtic and Gaelic folklore and is one of the twelve trees of the Celtic calendar. It was particularly associated with May Day (Beltane), when blossoming branches of hawthorn would be used for decorations at parties and rituals. Loved by witches and faeries alike, hawthorn makes a good magical ally, especially when we are going through times of grief and loss.

Hibiscus (*Hibiscus* spp.*)

This tropical shrub with its vibrantly colored flowers can be grown in containers for those with smaller gardens or limited space. Very high in vitamin C, tea made from the petals and sepals of this plant is full of antioxidant and anti-inflammatory properties and helps to regulate blood pressure.

Yet hibiscus also works powerfully on both emotional and magical levels: the flowers can help us become more passionate in all areas of our lives. Added to drinks or stirred into cake batters, dried hibiscus flowers will help draw love and emotional healing into our lives—including new romance, if that is what we are seeking. This beautiful plant is a great healing ally for past traumas, particularly

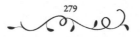

those of an emotional or sexual nature, and helps us move on to a healed and more grounded space.

Honeybush (*Cyclopia faboideae)*

This plant, native to the Eastern Cape region of South Africa, is actually related to rooibos, and its use in teas and other medicinal and beauty preparations has increased considerably over the past few years. High in vitamin C and antioxidants, it's an excellent tea for improving overall health and vitality—and as an added bonus, it's caffeine free!

Honeysuckle (*Lonicera* spp.*)*

There are many varieties of this beautifully fragrant plant with an unmistakeable fragrance; it's long been a part of traditional herbalism and mythology and was believed to avert evil powers and also ensure that cows gave good milk. When infused and used in teas, the flowers can be helpful for colds, coughs, and asthma. Emotionally, honeysuckle is a particularly powerful flower for creating a more balanced and joyful sense of self, for helping us let go of things that no longer serve us well and accept changes in our lives with grace and courage. If you want to get in touch with your inner divine powers, using honeysuckle will help you access this realm of possibility, true magic, and wisdom.

The flowers can be used fresh (this includes adding them to salads or sprinkling them over iced teas and desserts) or they can be dried for use in the cooler months. Please note that honeysuckle berries are poisonous and should not be consumed.

Hops (*Humulus lupulus*)

Not just for making beer, the flowers of this vine have been used medicinally for centuries in teas and tinctures for their antibacterial and antimicrobial properties. How-ever, the main benefit of hops is their mildly sedative and calming qualities. They have long been an ingredient for sleep and dream pillows and can also be used in teas to promote a restful and calm night. Tea made with hops is a powerful help for those of us who suffer from insomnia, particularly when the sleeplessness is linked to tension, fear, and anxiety.

Jasmine (*Jasminum officinale*)

I can still remember the first time I was taken out to a family dinner at a local Chinese restaurant—I was prob-ably about nine or ten; after the delicious meal, we were served tiny red and gold cups of delicate jasmine tea, as is traditional in the East, where it's used as a gentle digestive after meals. I was familiar with jasmine as a plant, of course, since my mom had a lot of it growing in the garden, but the

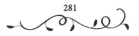

unmistakeable flavor and aroma was quite something else in tea form.

Jasmine is an absolute gift to those of us who seek more joy, peace, and abundance in our lives—and who doesn't? This tea brings us back to ourselves in a wonderfully simple and natural way, and this magical effect is enhanced when we add a few dried rose petals to our jasmine tea blend. It's also an excellent stress reliever on every level, so consider using jasmine tea for anxiety, anger, tension, and general depletion of body and spirit.

Juniper (*Juniperus communis*)

The berries of this small evergreen conifer have been used since ancient times. The Romans believed this tree conferred powerful protection, and in fact juniper trees are featured in many different legends, usually playing the role of guardian and safekeeper. The berries are also an essential part of the gin-making process and are used for other culinary purposes as well as being helpful for health issues such as coughs, lung infections, and cystitis. However, they should be used with caution by people with kidney problems and not at all during pregnancy. Dried berries can be added to teas and infusions; keep in airtight jars and do not store for more than six months, as after that the berries lose much of their flavor and potency.

Lady's Mantle (*Alchemilla* spp.*)

This ancient and healing herb is native to the mountains of Europe, Asia, and America and grows well in the damp, shady protection of woods and trees. It was believed in medieval times that dew collected from the leaves of this plant would preserve a woman's youth and beauty, as well as protect her from any malevolent forces. It was also sacred to the Virgin Mary, hence the name.

Lady's Mantle is, as its name would suggest, a particularly helpful healing plant for female issues, such as conditions of the uterus and breasts or problems with menstruation and menopause. The leaves can be used fresh or dried to make a tea that should be drunk for at least ten days before and during the onset of a period; it will also ease menopausal symptoms.

Lavender (*Lavender angustifolia*)

Probably one of the most popular all-round herbs, this fragrant beauty has been around for centuries and has a multitude of uses—culinary, health, beauty, and well-being. There are many species of lavender, some more highly scented than others, but all can be used in a similar way. For the purposes of herbal teas, I generally use the fresh (or dried) flowers rather than the leaves; it's a good idea to be fairly judicious in their use, too, since lavender is

283

a strong herb and too much of it can be a little overwhelming! For this reason, just a little of the herb is often used in conjunction with other herbs or even green or black tea.

Lavender tea is a wonderful remedy for insomnia, nervous tension and stress, and depression, and it also soothes and relieves headaches, indigestion, and colic. It's generally mild enough to be taken by just about anybody, but as it can be a uterine stimulant, it's best to avoid too much lavender during pregnancy.

Lemon (*Citrus limon*)

Is it a fruit? Is it a herb? Actually, it's both, and I, like so many others, could not function without a steady supply of lemons in my kitchen, bathroom cupboard, and herbal tea chest! All parts of this ancient fruit are full of natural vitamins, astringents, and alkalisers, and of course the fresh, bright flavor is quite irreplaceable. Lemon has anti-inflammatory and antibiotic properties, and it also helps lower blood pressure and cholesterol. It's widely used in preparations for coughs, colds, and flu, and a simple tea made with lemon slices, hot water, and honey is a wonderful way to start the day on a bright and healthy note.

All parts of the lemon can be used, either fresh or dried; this includes the blossoms and leaves, which make a good addition to teas and spicy foods. Lemon also partners well

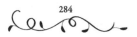

with other herbs, and of course is a longstanding companion for various green and black traditional teas.

Lemon Balm (*Melissa officinalis*)

This pretty and fragrant plant is a must-have in any herbal tea garden. The lemon-scented leaves make a refreshing and relaxing tea, helpful for calming stress and easing digestive problems. The aromatic leaves—which can be used fresh or dried—have a truly unforgettable and alluring fragrance, sweet and fresh at the same time. The fresh leaves make a delightful tea that is packed with all kinds of healing properties; lemon verbena is excellent for treating colds, asthma, fever, and digestive problems, particularly those related to nervous conditions, as it has a mild sedative and calming effect. Used magically, it can help remove old and negative patterns of thinking and bring about fresh and positive insight.

Lemongrass (*Cymbopogon citratus*)

Another herb generally used for culinary purposes, particularly in Far Eastern cooking, lemongrass is also powerful magically and is traditionally used for protection and removing negative forces, either from the body or the home. Lemongrass stems are quite tough but can be used whole when added to boiling liquids; alternatively, peel away the hard outer layers and finely chop the more tender

inner stems before adding them to teas, flavored waters, or desserts.

Lemongrass has calming, antidepressant, and sedative properties and can be used to ease painful joints, back-aches, and headaches. This herb was traditionally used to increase creativity and bring about greater mental clarity and focus. It also is said to strengthen psychic powers and can be used in magical recipes as a substitute for mugwort.

Avoid using lemongrass medicinally if you are pregnant or breastfeeding; the stems may irritate sensitive skin.

Linden (*Tilia europaea*)

Linden trees are a very familiar sight in Europe, where the flowers are traditionally brewed into tisanes, partic-ularly as a calming after-dinner drink that ensures good digestion and a peaceful night's sleep because of its mild sedative qualities, which help ease anxiety and tension. It's also used for treating high blood pressure, especially when stress related, and helps to reduce fatty deposits in blood vessels that can cause potentially dangerous healthy issues like heart attacks or strokes. Needless to say, this should not replace medical evaluation and treatment by health professionals.

In ancient lore and legend, linden is considered both magical and a protection against evil spirits and harmful

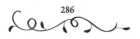

forces. The tree is sacred to the Virgin Mary, and shrines to her are often hung on its branches or trunks in Europe.

Linden can help us heal emotionally when we are going through times of pain, hurt, and heartbreak; drinking linden tea helps us reconnect with healthy and peaceful emotional energies and reminds us that we are always able to access the love and support of our great earth mother.

Marjoram (*Origanum majorana*)

Much more than just a delicious culinary herb, marjoram—rather like its close cousin oregano, which is a little strong and wilder in taste—is filled with all kinds of soothing and healing properties. It's a natural antispasmodic and antibacterial plant that can be used for digestive problems, nausea, colic, bloating, and respiratory issues.

Marjoram is also a powerfully protective herb and was used to ward off evil intent and dark forces during the Middle Ages. However, even if that is not really a problem for you, this herbal tea will help with feelings of anxiety, fear, restlessness, and nightmares. Like oregano, it's a symbol of happiness, too, and sipping this tea not only lifts our spirits but gives us new vision and hope.

Meadowsweet (*Filipendula* spp.)

This fragrant herb with its little almond-scented flowers is much loved by bees. The whole plant can be used for its

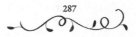

astringent and anti-inflammatory properties, particularly for arthritis, rheumatism, pain, and digestive complaints.

Meadowsweet was regarded by the Druids as a sacred herb and often used in love spells and wedding ceremonies. It helps heal and remove emotional blocks that are preventing us from moving on and forward with our lives.

Mint (*Mentha* spp.)

An essential in the herbal tea garden, although it must be planted in its own space or pot given its rampant tendency to spread and take over other plants! It's a truly ancient herb that has been used for various purification rituals down the centuries, from the Greek gods on Mount Olympus to the temple of King Solomon. This summer herb can also be dried for use throughout the year since it is one of the herbs that retains excellent flavor when dried, owing to its high levels of volatile oils.

Peppermint (*Mentha piperita*) is the most widely used of the mint family; it's an old tea remedy for digestive problems of all kinds, including pain, bloating, and nausea. Mint is also a calmative herb, ideal for insomnia, anxiety disorders, and times of stress. Peppermint tea is also said to be an aid for divination and prophetic dreams. It helps to clear and lift blocked or stagnant emotional energy and brings us greater clarity and energy, especially as regards the best use of our purpose and gifts here on this earth.

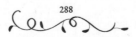

Avoid drinking peppermint tea for periods longer than eight weeks at a time; large quantities should also be avoided in pregnant or breastfeeding women and can also sometimes aggravate acid reflux disease, or heartburn. Peppermint is not recommended for use with children under the age of five.

Motherwort (*Leonurus cardiaca*)

This protective herb, a member of the mint family, has been used since ancient times as a treatment during childbirth and also to help menstrual problems. Because of its calming effect, it is soothing for times of nervous stress and exhaustion, especially those causing insomnia and a racing heart or elevated blood pressure. However, as it is a uterine stimulant, it should not be taken during pregnancy. Use motherwort in teas when you want to experience clear and lucid dreams or for divination purposes.

Mugwort (*Artemisia vulgaris*)

This is one of the most ancient and magical of all herbs and is traditionally associated with protection against evil spirits and negative energies of all kinds. This plant spreads easily in the garden, so is best planted in pots; it should be kept well-trimmed. The harvested leaves and roots are both used in medicinal and magical applications and can be used fresh or dried. Mugwort helps with menstrual problems, indigestion, fevers, and sleeplessness.

This herb is linked to moon energies, and a tea made with mugwort leaves will help you dream more clearly and prophetically. It can also be used during ceremonies or rituals invoking the spirit world. This is also a powerfully protective herb for working against negative forces or entities; mugwort can guide us to better and safer paths for body and spirit.

Please note that mugwort should not be taken when pregnant.

Nasturtium (*Tropaeolum majus*)

This bright and happy plant is a big favorite in gardens, and understandably so: not only does it add a burst of brilliant color, but it's a truly multipurpose herb—seeds, flowers, and leaves all have medicinal and culinary uses. Very easy to grow, they are happy in containers too, and the trailing varieties are delightful in hanging baskets.

Best used fresh, the leaves and flowers are extremely high in vitamin C and strengthen the immune system as well as have antiseptic and digestive properties. They can be used to make tisanes or, chopped up and sprinkled, on jugs of iced tea or as a garnish for baked goods.

Nasturtiums are full of positive vibes and promote happiness, something easy to understand when you look at their sunny, open blooms. Add nasturtium to tea when you need to clear away some dark clouds of mind or mood and find a brighter outlook.

Nettle (*Urtica dioica*)

Not called stinging nettle for nothing, so please use caution—and wear long sleeves and gloves—when harvesting any part of this plant. Actually, this is an extremely valuable herb; although in much of the Northern Hemisphere it is simply viewed as a weed, nettles have all kinds of therapeutic and culinary uses (nettle soup or pesto are quite delicious). The plant is very high in both minerals and vitamins.

Nettle tea, which can be made from fresh leaves and flowers or those that you have dried for the winter months, stimulates circulation, treats viral infections, and helps regulate blood sugar levels. It's a traditional blood-cleansing remedy and is helpful for arthritis, gout, and other joint-related issues; it also helps strengthen hair and nails and keep them in peak condition. Try using a few cups of cool nettle tea as a final rinse after shampooing your hair.

Nettle has always been a powerful ally of green witches, a reminder of the wild possibilities we contain within our beings and the potential we have for growth and change. Nettle is a strong herb that allows us to become who we are unapologetically and exercise our right to create healthy personal boundaries.

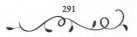

Nutmeg (*Myristica fragrans*)

This tropical plant's seed gives us two spices: the inner spice pod (nutmeg) is covered by a network of mace. Warming and fragrant, nutmeg makes an excellent addition to herbal teas, although it should always be used with discretion as it is potent, and too much can potentially be toxic.

Nutmeg is traditionally used for digestive issues such as nausea, flatulence, and stomach cramps, but in the East it is also reputed to be helpful for joint and muscular issues such as rheumatism. (And it was also reputed to be an aphrodisiac, but that I can't confirm!) If possible, buy whole nutmegs (with the mace still attached) and store in an airtight jar in a cool, dark place—grate a little of the nutmeg (and mace) fresh, as and when needed; of course, you can easily buy ground nutmeg too, but in general it loses some of its bright pungency when stored too long.

Oatstraw (*Avena sativa*)

This may not be an ingredient you already have on your kitchen shelf, but oatstraw is relatively easy to grow. Teas made with dried oatstraw have been used for centuries as a tonic and to build up immunity, as well as for arthritic pain, skin problems, thyroid issues, depression and anxiety, colds and flu, and menopausal problems (oats can reduce oestrogen deficiency).

Oats can be dried and tied into bundles for use in teas and other applications; this is a powerful grounding plant that reminds us of the need to let go of expectations, fear, and questioning, and simply be quiet, fully in the moment. Use this ancient herbal remedy when you need to bring back some childlike joy and vitality to your being and discover a new enthusiasm for your life.

Please note that the regular oats we are familiar with are not the same and cannot be used for teas.

Olive Leaf (*Olea europea*)

We are all familiar with the olive, both as berry and oil, used as food and medicine—but some of us may not be used to olive leaves being used for tea purposes too. Olives have been sacred to many cultures over the centuries, but it is only recently that the leaves of the olive tree have been found to contain many amazing antiviral and antibacterial properties, in addition to helping regulate blood pressure, ease fatigue, and lower blood sugar levels.

On a spiritual level, olive leaf can be both comforting and uplifting when we are feeling despairing and totally exhausted by life. Teas can be made by pouring just-boiled water over fresh leaves and sprigs; they can also be dried for use but are less effective that way. You may need to add some honey or cinnamon to make the tea a little more palatable.

293

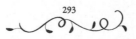

Orange (*Citrus sinensis*)

This much-loved fruit is truly versatile: the juice, rind, and flesh can be added to various tea blends and are suitable for both hot and iced beverages of all kinds. Dried orange peel can be stored in small jars and used all year round; it's also excellent when mixed with other citrus such as lemon rind/zest. Orange has magical qualities of love, friendship, cleansing, creativity, and success. Use dried orange peel as a substitute for neroli in magical formulas.

Oregano (*Oregano vulgare*)

A native herb of the Mediterranean region and a close relative of marjoram, although oregano is stronger and wilder in taste and scent. In Greece the name translates as "joy of the mountain," and it is an indispensable herb in Greek cooking (and in mine). In ancient times it was believed that if oregano was found growing on graves, it meant that the dead were happy in the afterlife. The goddess Venus grew this fragrant herb in her garden, and it was linked to beauty and faithfulness in love.

The leaves and flowers can be used fresh or dried—they retain their scent and flavor very well. The list of the therapeutic uses of this plant is long: it's warming, antiviral, antibacterial, relieves inflammation and pain, and eases painful stomach cramps and flatulence. The high levels of thymol in this plant make it a natural remedy for lung and respiratory issues, as well as toothaches, sore joints, and rheumatism. It's also helpful for nervous conditions and can calm frayed nerves. However, it's best to make limited use of this herb if you are pregnant or breastfeeding or with children under the age of seven.

Parsley (*Petroselinum crispum*)

Probably one of the best known of the culinary herbs, parsley (in either the curly or flat-leaved form) is also useful for herbal teas—although personally I am not a big fan of the taste. However, this herb is packed with vitamins and iron, and it has been used since ancient times to treat everything from arthritis to bladder infections and chest ailments to blood pressure problems. It's considered an excellent cure for hangovers and overindulgences of any kind.

Parsley taken as a tea, either alone or added to other herbs such as lemon or thyme, makes an excellent detox or diuretic and boosts the system on every level. However, it should always be taken in fairly moderate amounts and not over a long period of time.

Passionflower (*Passiflora incarnata*)

A truly beautiful and dynamic plant, the name derives from the last days and suffering of Jesus Christ. Planted in your garden, passionflower will attract droves of birds,

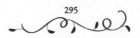

bees, wasps, and butterflies to its colorful blooms. The entire plant can be used to make teas and tinctures, and it has been used medicinally by Native Americans in both the North and South Hemispheres for centuries to treat disorders such as skin, blood, and circulatory problems.

Passionflower is also a gentle sedative, used to calm anxiety and persistent fearful or intrusive thoughts, and can help alleviate mild depression. Passionflower relaxes us on all levels—and it is only when we are truly still that we can find real rest, as well as opening ourselves to expanded joy and possibilities; this enables us to become truly creative in whatever field we choose and find new self-confidence in what we choose to bring into the world. Use passionflower when you want to go on inward journeys of discovery and for prayer and meditation work.

Pine (*Pinus* spp.)

This beautiful, tall evergreen (which can reach heights of up to 100 feet) is instantly recognizable both by its appearance and the distinctive, fresh aroma of its needles. It was mentioned in Roman mythology and is also one of the sacred trees of the Irish chieftains. A tea made of pine needles can help clear and clarify mind and emotions and create a more positive emotional state, especially when we are going through periods of grief, remorse, and self-doubt.

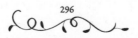

Primrose (*Primula vulgaris)*

The old meaning of this pretty plant's name is "first rose," which refers to the fact that the delightful pale blossoms of this plant make their first appearance in early spring. In medieval days they were used to make love potions and were also considered a remedy for gout, rheumatism, and headaches. These days a tisane made from the leaves and flowers (preferably fresh) has gentle sedative effects and as such is good for anxiety and insomnia. The flowers can also be used (either fresh or crystallized) in salads or sprinkled over iced teas and other cold beverages or on baked goods. However, it should be noted that working with this plant can cause a form of contact dermatitis in certain individuals.

Raspberry (*Rubus idaeus)*

We are all familiar with this bright and flavorful little fruit that is so delicious in desserts, jellies, jams, and baked goods, but the leaves of this rambling plant have also been used to make herbal tea for centuries. Raspberry leaves are loaded with vitamins, minerals, and antioxidants and can be used as a tonic, digestive herb, or diuretic. A raspberry leaf infusion was often traditionally drunk during the last few weeks of pregnancy to strengthen and tone the uterus before giving birth; for this reason, the tea should not be

taken in the early months of pregnancy as it can stimulate the uterus.

On a magical level, raspberry leaves and juice are wonderful for spell and ritual work involving protection and increased stamina and mental powers. Sacred to the goddess Aphrodite, drink this tea when you want to ramp up your love life on every level!

Rooibos (*Aspalathus linearis*)

Although rooibos (red bush) is only grown in its native country, South Africa, it is known internationally and available just about everywhere. Part of the fynbos family of plants, the needlelike green leaves turn red when processed and fermented. The tea has a rich, smoky flavor and is high in antioxidants while also being low in both tannin and caffeine. It would be virtually impossible to list all the healing qualities that have been linked to this mineral-rich herbal tea, but some of the main ones include improving skin conditions, weight loss, improved digestion, bone density, heart health, and helping with diabetes.

Infusions of rooibos are used in just about everything from baked goods to skincare products. Personally, I and many others find the flavor a little overpowering on its own, so often recipes and commercial produced teas will combine rooibos with other flowers and herbs; a particular favorite is rooibos and chamomile. Rooibos infusions also

work well in iced teas, where their sunny flavor seems to be particularly appropriate.

Rose (*Rosa* spp.)

Probably the most recognised, loved, and beautiful flower in the world since ancient times, roses are the source of many magical myths and legends—many of them true! Dried or fresh rose petals are wonderful when added to tea and also form part of many commercial tea blends, both herbal and traditional. If you are planning on growing and using your own roses for this purpose, you will need to choose highly scented varieties and also ensure that no noxious chemicals are used in their cultivation. The roses you can buy from the florist are not usually suitable as they generally lack fragrance, and also there is no way of ascertaining how they were cultivated.

The physical and emotional healing properties of roses are almost too many to be listed: however, they include stress, anxiety, menstrual problems, indigestion, urinary tract infections, and insomnia. Perhaps most of all, rose reminds us that we are worthy of nurture and self-care, and never more so than when we are feeling alone, unloved, or ignored. Simply adding a few dried rose petals to a cup of boiling water with a little honey and sipping this mixture slowly will immediately calm and soothe the most anxious mind. Rosehips, too, make a wonderful addition to herbal

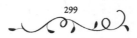

teas or drinks in their own right; cooked into a syrup with honey and lemon, this mixture can be kept to drink throughout the winter months, as it is a powerful immune booster against colds and flu. Simply add a few spoons of rosehip syrup to a mug of hot water and sip as needed.

Rosemary (*Rosmarinus officinalis*)

Few of us are not familiar with this highly aromatic herb that has literally hundreds of uses in the kitchen, for healing, and for just about anything where we need its warming, uplifting flavor and fragrance. The strong volatile oils in rosemary mean that it stands up well to drying and does not lose flavor in the process, so either fresh or dried leaves can be used in herbal teas and more—with one caveat: with rosemary less is more as it is such a powerful herb.

This herb is a wonderful tonic for both body and mind; it cleanses and oxygenates the blood and organs and also works to ease and improve digestive issues of all kinds. As far as the emotions are concerned, rosemary is truly magic—it helps lift and stabilise low moods and anxiety and is ideal for use when we are feeling uninspired, lacking in focus, and unable to concentrate effectively. Rosemary combines well with other herbs, particularly lavender, and a tea combining these two herbs is a beautiful way to unwind and relax both body and mind.

Rue (*Ruta graveolens*)

I was actually unsure as to whether to include this herb here. Personally, I find its scent both appealing and repelling at the same time, but it is a herb that has been used for hundreds of years, particularly for its mystical and protection powers. It's also credited with improving both eyesight and creativity: both Michaelangelo and Leonardo da Vinci claimed that rue helped them create their famous works of art.

The leaves and stems can be used in infusions and teas—but you will probably have to add other herbs or honey to help mask the bitter and pungent taste. Apparently, the tea works on improving the circulation, lowering blood pressure, and regulating menstruation, but since I can't stand the taste, I have no personal experience of this. A few cautionary notes: don't use rue if you are pregnant, and as it can be toxic in large doses, always use it with discretion. Some people also develop skin irritations when handling rue leaves, so it might be wise to wear gloves when picking the plant.

Sage (*Salvia officinalis*)

Many of us are more familiar with the use of sage in cooking, where it has a long and noble history, but perhaps are less aware that sage can be used to make wonderful

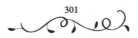

herbal teas and other beverages. There are many kinds of this pungent and aromatic herb, and they have a number of medicinal, culinary, and magical uses, but ordinary garden sage is the one generally available. White sage has been used for centuries in purification rituals but has been over-cultivated in recent years, so should be used with restraint.

When used in tea, sage has a strong but lovely flavor and contains so much medicine for both body and soul. It is an excellent nerve tonic, helping with stress, exhaustion, insomnia, and general debilitation of the nerves, as it gently promotes mental relaxation and clears negative energy.

It's also great at supporting digestion, helping with colds, flu, and other feverish conditions, and as a microbial agent can also be used for mouth and teeth problems and gum disease. However, high doses of sage should not be taken during pregnancy, and it should be avoided if you suffer from epilepsy.

Schisandra (*Schisandra chinensis*)

This climbing vine with clusters of red berries is native to northern China, Russia, and Korea; it's an important part of traditional Chinese medicine and is considered to be important for balancing the qi, or spirit. This plant is an adaptogen and helps improve stamina and vitality while strengthening and supporting the various systems and

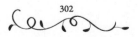

organs of the body. It helps to relieve low and depressed states of mind and gives us greater focus and renewed purpose in our lives.

Teas and infusions made from the berries can be drunk hot or cold and should ideally be taken on a daily basis for at least a few weeks in order to see good results. For a milder tea, this berry can be combined with other herbs like hibiscus or oatstraw, as a tea made from the berries alone can be quite stimulating for those who are a little depleted or frail physically, for whatever reason.

Self-Heal (*Prunella vulgaris*)

A small herb with little fuzzy purple flowers much loved by bees! Both the leaves and flowers are edible and can be used either dried or fresh for teas. Antibiotic and antioxidant in nature, self-heal has been around for centuries. As the name suggests, it is excellent for easing the discomfort of colds, flu, and fevers.

However, this is also a highly magical plant and is used for enchanted rituals and the creation of significant change in our lives on any level. We often think we are small and lacking in any real power, but self-heal gently reminds us of all that we are, and can be, in this world.

Skullcap (*Scutellaria*)

Many species of this little flower are found throughout Europe and North America, where it has been used extensively for various medical conditions such as insomnia, headaches, indigestion, and stomach cramps. It's also helpful for treating anxiety and depression, and both the leaves and flowers can be dried and used in teas and infusions. However, some sources suggest this herb is best dispensed and used under the guidance of a trained herbalist.

St. John's Wort (*Hypericum perforatum*)

A truly magical and healing herb on so many levels, it's been known and used since ancient times. *Wort* is an Anglo-Saxon word meaning "medicinal herb." (It was named for St. John, as the flowers bloom around the time of his beheading, June 24.) It's credited with magic powers and taking those who ingest it on amazing journeys both physically and psychologically. It was also believed to have the power to exorcise demonic spirits and raise ghosts to communicate with us.

Both the leaves and flowers can be used and contain anti-inflammatory and antibiotic properties; this herb is also helpful for neuralgia and painful joints. However, it's as a natural antidepressant and anxiolytic that St. John's wort is primarily used, and it is very effective in treating these all-too-common conditions. It's also helpful for PMS and psychological problems around menopause.

However, because it is a powerful herb, it should only be taken internally under medical supervision; thus, only very small quantities should be used in teas and infusions. Some people find they become more sensitive to sunlight or develop skin rashes when using the herb. It should be avoided by pregnant or breastfeeding women. It also goes without saying that if you are taking any existing medication for issues such as depression or anxiety, you should discuss this with your healthcare professional before using the herb.

Star Anise (*Illicium verum*)

Native to both China and Vietnam, this beautiful spice with its star-shaped seeds is used in recipes for pork, chicken, and soups such as Vietnamese pho. A few of these seeds with their sweet, anise-like flavor can be added to teas and other beverages; they are used in the East for pain relief and to ease coughing.

Powerful for creating wish magic, star anise increases intuition and helps us purify our spirits to access deeper and more aware states of being.

Strawberry (*Fragaria* spp.*)

Probably one of the most-loved berries, they are sacred to the goddesses Freya and Aphrodite as well as the Virgin Mary, so are linked with protection, fertility, luck, and love. Obviously the berries can be sliced and used in chilled tea drinks of all kinds, as well as in baking, but the leaves can also be added to teas or dried and then crumbled and used in blends.

Tarragon (*Artemisia dracunculus*)

There are two varieties of this plant, French and Russian tarragon. French tarragon's fresh and light aniseed flavor is the preferred one of the two and is extensively used in cooking and in the making of preserves such as tarragon vinegar, which is a delightful way of adding this herb's flavor to salads, sauces, and fish dishes.

However, tarragon is also a medicinal herb and can be used in teas or infusions for digestive problems, insomnia, and as a general tonic for the whole system. The leaves can be used fresh or dried, as they retain their flavor well.

Thyme (*Thymus vulgaris*)

I just love thyme and would never be without it, either in my kitchen or bathroom cabinet—it is such a useful and delightful herb! Although there are many varieties of thyme, just the regular culinary thyme will suit most appli-

cations; however, if you can get hold of lemon thyme, I would suggest you grow that too, as it is particularly good in teas and baked goods. (Thyme dries well and keeps its bright, characteristic flavor, so either fresh or dried leaves can be used interchangeably.) And don't forget the pretty little flowers, which can also be used as needed!

Thyme is an antiseptic and antimicrobial herb, which makes it ideal for treating problems of the respiratory system as well as being good for digestive issues of all kinds, including bloating and diarrhoea. If you suffer from tension headaches or migraines, thyme will provide gentle relief. And thyme is known for its uplifting properties, encouraging a sense of optimism and hope when we feel totally depleted; it gives us courage and a sense of new possibility. Avoid taking large amounts of thyme if you are pregnant or breastfeeding.

Turmeric (*Curcuma longa*)

This member of the ginger family with its bright golden color and slightly musky aroma has been cultivated for over 2,000 years and was used in ancient Persian rituals of sun worship. Today it is still widely used as both a culinary spice and a medicine, and turmeric is becoming increasingly popular as its many health benefits have been uncovered, in particular its chemical component, curcumin, which is linked to blood pressure reduction, memory

improvement, easing of arthritis/joint pain, and the lessening of depressive symptoms.

Although the fresh root is sometimes available, turmeric is usually found in its ground, dried form; it can be added to teas (in moderation, as it can be bitter if used in excess). This spice should be avoided if you have gall bladder disease, disorders of the blood/clotting issues, endometriosis, and cancers of the female reproductive system.

Valerian (*Valerian officinalis)*

This tall and upright plant was mentioned by Hippocrates, the father of modern medicine, so it has a long and honorable history. Valerian is a powerful relaxant for the nervous system and as such can be used to treat insomnia, stress, or anxiety. However, it should not be used in conjunction with other antidepressants; if you are in doubt, consult your healthcare provider for advice.

The roots (either fresh or dried) can be used for teas and tinctures; however, it has to be said that dried valerian root is not particularly appetising in taste or aroma, so is generally better if combined with other herbs or sweetened with a little honey.

This herb was traditionally used for Samhain and Yule festivals and rituals and for the casting of both love spells and those that protect against evil or negative entities and bad dreams. Valerian invites us to rest, let go of our fears

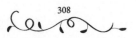

and self-doubt, and allow ourselves to truly experience our emotions without censure or blame.

Vanilla (*Vanilla planifolia*)

Not a herb and not really a spice either, vanilla is arguably one of the most recognised scents in the world—which of us doesn't know its sweet warmth in desserts and baked goods? But vanilla beans actually come from the fruit pods of an orchid and are generally sold dried; you can also buy vanilla extract (please, please not cheap commercial essence, which contains no value at all). For tea purposes, I suggest you buy the dried pods and carefully scrape out a few seeds (they are very potent) as and when you need them. The pods should be kept in a sealed glass container. The seeds can also be added to sugar or honey, which then is great used in baked goods or to sweeten teas and other beverages.

Vanilla has mild pain-relieving and antiseptic properties; however, its main gifts to us are its ability to help disperse and relieve stress and anxiety and bring about a sense of positivity and hope. Vanilla is nontoxic and nonirritant, but remember that less is more when using it as both its flavor and aroma are very strong.

Vervain (*Verbena officinalis*)

Not to be confused with lemon verbena, this ancient and healing herb was widely used by Native Americans as a tonic and remedy for all kinds of ailments such as fevers, coughs, colds, and digestive complaints. But it is the magical qualities of this herb that are truly exceptional: vervain can help us find our calm center and balance our emotions, helping clear away mental blocks and negativity. Widely used for divination and spellwork at Samhain, this herb allows us to look beyond the obvious and travel to places of enchantment and magic. For this reason, it's also quite a powerful herb, so should be used in moderation; too much can cause nausea and other digestive issues.

Violet (*Viola odorata*)

I remember my mother had some patches of these dainty flowers with their unmistakeable and haunting fragrance growing in a quiet and shady corner of her garden; even as a little girl I was drawn to them, and their nostalgic scent has made them a favorite for centuries. The humble violet was loved by the ancient Greeks and first recorded as a medicinal plant in the first century CE. Violet teas and tinctures were used in the Middle East, North Africa, and Europe, particularly France, where they remain a favorite to this day.

Used as a medicinal tea, violet leaves, flowers, and roots are soothing and healing for coughs, flu, sinusitis, and sore throats. The flowers are beautiful when used as decoration for baked goods and desserts and may be crystallized for this purpose. Fragrances often include violets for their sweetly comforting and uplifting effect, and this will also be found when drinking the tea. This pretty plant also has the ancient name of heartsease, which seems entirely appropriate given its gentle and uplifting nature.

Willow (*Salix* spp.)

An incredibly beautiful and graceful tree with soft and swooping branches, willow has been loved and revered for centuries in many different cultures. It is a sacred tree to all major religions and is also one of the thirteen magical trees of the Celtic year; many ancient stories celebrated the ancient mystery of this enchanting plant. There are many species of willow, found in most parts of the world; all of them die back in fall and are born again in spring, echoing the spirit of regeneration that is at the heart of willow's eternal magic.

Medicinally, willow is the source of salicylic acid (the core ingredient in aspirin), and the medical uses of this plant have been documented since ancient times. In addition to its pain-relieving qualities, willow is also anti-inflammatory and can be used to ease joint and muscle

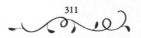

problems; it's also an antiseptic herb and useful for fevers and winter conditions like colds and flu.

Teas made from the chopped leaves of willow have strong emotional healing properties: they help with painful and intrusive feelings, offer protection from negativity (either from within or from outside sources), and teach us to be flexible and accept change with grace and fortitude. This is particularly true when we are going through periods of grief or loss that we find difficult to accept.

Yarrow (*Achillea millefolium*)

This ancient herb, which grows prolifically in Europe, North America, and Asia, has long been considered to have both magical and sacred associations. It was used by the Druids to read weather signs and portents and was also said to confer protection against evil or negative forces.

Fresh or dried leaves and flowers can be used to make teas and infusions that are particularly effective for fevers and inflammatory conditions. It should always be taken in moderation, though, and not when pregnant.

Yerba Santa (*Eriodictyon californicum*)

As the name suggests, this shiny dark-green shrub is native to California as well as Oregon and parts of northern Mexico. It grows in wild, dry, hot desert and mountain areas and has been a traditional healing herb of the indig-

enous peoples of these areas for thousands of years. The name *yerba santa* means "holy herb," which suggests that it had many uses on both the physical and spiritual levels. Medically, the herb has been used for lung and respiratory complaints, as an aid for digestive complaints, and for cleansing the body with its powerful antimicrobial action.

The leaves, which can be brewed into a tea or added to blends and infusions, are also excellent at calming the mind and easing racing, anxious thoughts; we become quiet and still, open to the moment, and for this reason the herb has been used for meditation practices and to undertake shamanic journeys. It can shift our consciousness into a different realm, one in which we truly see beyond everyday seeing and can access what lies beneath everyday awareness.

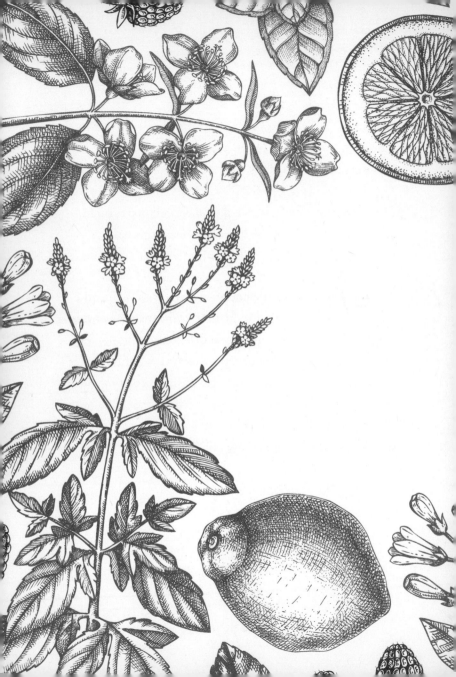

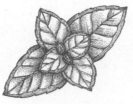

CONCLUSION

I hope this little book has served as a useful and inspirational introduction to the magical world of tea, in all its many and delicious facets. As you travel on your own tea journey, I trust you will find it an enchanted, healing, and sacred one; the ideas contained in this book are really intended to be stepping stones along a path that ultimately leads to a garden tea party that is steeped in green magic and moonlight!

Pour your tea. Sit a while. You are welcome here; you are loved. There is nothing you have to do, nothing that needs to be accomplished. Sit and drink your tea, knowing all is as it should be.

Breathe and dream deep. Enchantment and peace are yours, now and always.

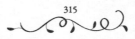

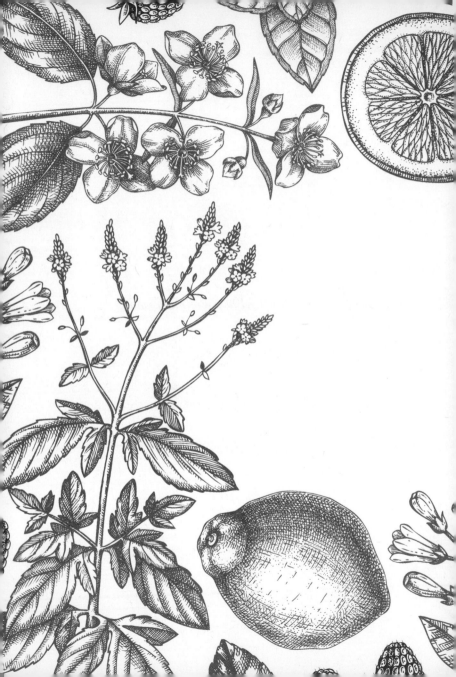

BIBLIOGRAPHY

This is a short list of books that have been a help and inspiration to me on my herbal journey.

Bremness, Lesley. *The Complete Book of Herbs*. London: Dorling Kindersley, 1988.

Franklin, Anna. *The Hearth Witch's Kitchen Herbal*. Woodbury, MN: Llewellyn Worldwide, 2019.

Hesse, Eelco. *Tea: The Eyelids of Bodhidharma*. Dorset: Prism Press, 1982.

Johnson, Cait. *Witch in the Kitchen*. Rochester, VT: Destiny Books, 2001.

Kynes, Sandra. *Sea Magic*. Woodbury, MN: Llewellyn Worldwide, 2015.

McVicar, Jekka. *Jekka's Complete Herb Book*. London: Kyle Cathie Limited, 1994.

Miernowska, Marysia. *The Witch's Herbal Apothecary*. Beverly, MA: Fair Winds Press, 2020.

Morishita, Noriko. *The Wisdom of Tea*. London: Allen and Unwin, 2020.

Murphy-Hiscock, Arin. *The Witch's Book of Self-Care*. Avon, MA: Adams Media, 2018.

Nickerson, Brittany Wood. *Recipes from the Herbalist's Kitchen*. North Adams, MA: Storey Publishing, 2017.

Ortiz, Elizabeth Lambert. *The Encyclopedia of Herbs, Spices, and Flavorings*. London: Dorling Kindersley, 1992.

Perrakis, Athena. *The Book of Blessings and Rituals*. Beverly, MA: Fair Winds Press, 2019.

Reader's Digest Farmhouse Cookery. London: Reader's Digest Association, 1980.

Roberts, Margaret. *Herbal Teas for Healthy Living*. Cape Town: Random Struik, 2008.